Practicing Psychoanalysis in Israel

Gabriela Mann's book explores the work of an Israeli psychoanalyst who encounters the trauma and tragedy of Israelis living in an environment saturated with existential anxieties and threats to their well-being.

This work offers clinical materials that illustrate the possibility of expansion of the mind through a spiritual dimension in psychoanalysis. The main theme focuses on transcending from a narrow perspective to a broad compassionate view by uncovering the interconnectedness between seemingly different phenomena. This cultivates the patients' ability to free themselves from past and contemporary trauma. Drawing on Kohut, Bion, and Winnicott, as well as from Buddhist thinking, *Seeing Through Blindness* describes the transformation of archaic narcissism, usually concerned with individual goals, to mature narcissism which strives for a supra-individual perspective. The reader is invited to choose among the chapters that describe splits in the self, paradoxes of belonging, perpetrators and victims, perversion, and selfobject needs at times of threat and bereavement.

The book offers new ways of thinking about trauma in a troubled world for all psychoanalysts and psychoanalytic psychotherapists.

Gabriela Mann, PhD, is a training psychoanalyst, former Tel Aviv Institute of Contemporary Psychoanalysis chairperson, and faculty member of the Tel Aviv Medical School Psychotherapy Program and of Human Spirit – Psychoanalytic-Buddhist Training Program.

Evolutions in Psychoanalysis Book Series
DANIEL GOLDIN AND MELVIN BRONSTEIN Series Editors

Under the editorship of Melvin Bronstein and Daniel Goldin, the Evolutions in Psychoanalysis book series provides a shared space for writers who are eager to revisit formative psychoanalytical ideas in often innovative new ways. The word 'evolve' literally means 'to unroll', and the contemporary use of the latter term suggests that something new can be revealed through a process of incremental unravelling. As a definition of both the aspirations of this series and of psychoanalysis itself, this understanding exemplifies the possibility that one can take apart by creating and create by taking apart.

The volumes in this series do not represent a particular school of psychoanalytic thought, but rather comprise and encourage new voices from all schools and spaces – across time and geographical location – in the knowledge that brilliant thinkers and ideas can emerge from unforeseen places. The series does also encompass the editors' interests in how contemporary psychoanalysis intersects with society and culture at large; differing analyses of the micro-processes that take place in clinical encounters; and the influence of other disciplines – such as philosophy and infant-research – upon the field of psychoanalysis, and welcomes contributions to these and other topics.

Of critical importance to the formation of this series is its aspiration to foreground voices from marginalized ethnic groups, for the vitality and creativity they offer which is so necessary to the field, and to continue in the direction of redress and repair for the omissions and exclusions of the past.

Practicing Psychoanalysis in Israel
Seeing Through Blindness
Gabriela Mann

For more information about this series, please visit: www.routledge.com/Evolutions-in-Psychoanalysis-Book-Series/book-series/EVIPS

Practicing Psychoanalysis in Israel

Seeing Through Blindness

Gabriela Mann

Routledge
Taylor & Francis Group
LONDON AND NEW YORK

Designed cover image: Itamar Mann, Haifa 2023

First published in English 2025
by Routledge
4 Park Square, Milton Park, Abingdon, Oxon, OX14 4RN

and by Routledge
605 Third Avenue, New York, NY 10158

Routledge is an imprint of the Taylor & Francis Group, an informa business

First published in Hebrew by Resling Publishing house 2022

Library of Congress Cataloging-in-Publication Data
A catalog record for this book has been requested

ISBN: 978-1-032-58273-3 (hbk)
ISBN: 978-1-032-58275-7 (pbk)
ISBN: 978-1-003-44938-6 (ebk)

DOI: 10.4324/9781003449386

Typeset in Times New Roman
by Apex CoVantage, LLC

In loving memory of my parents, Rosel and Kurt Kanowitz, who found refuge and a new beginning in Israel

Contents

Acknowledgments

This book is the product of several years of work. Its completion was made possible through the assistance and encouragement of friends and colleagues. I am grateful to Professor Aner Govrin of Bar Ilan University, Senior Editor at Resling Publishing/Psychoanalysis Tel Aviv, who suggested that I write the Hebrew edition. This edition, *Seeing Through Blindness: On the Expansion of the Mind in Psychoanalysis*, was published in 2022. I am thankful for the support provided by Joe Lichtenberg, whom I met in Israel and later in the United States. He invited me to contribute to *Psychoanalytic Inquiry*, and this is how three of the chapters – Chapters, 4, 8, and 10 – were first published. I am also thankful to the Editorial Board of *The International Journal of Psychoanalytic Self Psychology* and *Psychoanalysis, Self and Context* for publishing papers whose first versions I presented at self psychology international conferences. This is how Chapter 3 was first published in the *International Journal of Psychoanalytic Self Psychology*. Carol Levin, whom I met at several conferences, encouraged me to submit an English edition to the *Psychoanalytic Inquiry Book series*, to which I added the "war chapter" (Chapter 1). I thank Carol for that encouragement and for introducing me to Daniel Goldin. I am most grateful to Daniel Goldin for welcoming my manuscript and assisting me throughout the publication process. Many thanks to Dan Gilon for his patience and effort in translating sometimes complex materials from Hebrew to English and to Simon P. Watmough for his incisive editing of the manuscript.

I also want to express my sincere appreciation to three people who had a major impact on my professional life: Yolanda Gampel, Neville Symington, and Raanan Kulka. Each draws from philosophic sources that transcend the main streams of psychoanalytic thinking. Yolanda is informed by Taoist concepts; Neville was informed by Christian and Zen mystics, and

Raanan is informed by Buddhist teachings. Yolanda, Neville, and Raanan inspired me for many years and informed my psychoanalytic thinking in many ways. Yolanda Gampel, a mental mentor for me, helped me to cultivate a psychoanalytic perspective on social violence. Neville Symington was one of my supervisors and a close friend, promoting my conviction to moral courage and helping patients to cultivate their inner freedom. Raanan Kulka plays a substantial role in my professional life. The many hours we spent talking taught me how to think about the spiritual aspects of psychoanalysis and help patients transcend their suffering. I am indebted to him for his intellectual and empathic support.

Finally, I wish to thank my children Itamar, Eytan, and Daniel, and their partners Shira, Noa, and Ayala, all of whom encouraged me to take on this project and stood beside me at every stage. They are my intellectual allies and closest friends. Above all, I am thankful to Kenneth Mann, my most careful reader and loving life partner. I could not have completed this book without his support.

Figures

Introduction

Gabriela Mann, PhD

I am preparing this book for publishing in the midst of a major catastrophe that we, Israelis, are presently experiencing. The war that erupted as a result of the attack on Israeli citizens and others in southern Israel on October 7, 2023, caused a collapse of the fundamental feeling of safety in one's home and a loss of confidence in Israel's resilience. We met the gods of cruelty and mercilessness. We feel misled by our government. And yet, at the same time, the human spirit prevails in many ways: thousands of people, young and old, volunteer and support the families of the kidnapped, the soldiers, and their families. They help the uprooted who lost their homes and live in temporary housing without knowing when it will be safe enough to return. Many are devoted to providing the injured in hospitals with a humane presence and needed supplies. Thousands of men and women attend demonstrations on a regular basis to protest the seeming collapse of effective government. This country is fighting for its democracy and sanity. At the same time, there is a deep concern among many of us about the fate of the citizens of Gaza, too many of whom have been killed, or whose homes have been destroyed, and who suffer from an insufficient supply of food and medical care. Presently, as I write, not enough has been done to address this humanitarian disaster.

This book is about how psychoanalysis in Israel contends with the human tragedies that are inherent in Israeli life, the present war included, and how psychoanalysts cultivate a human spirit in these circumstances. Its focal point is the transformation of the traumatic to the tragic. This transformation occurs at the fine line that separates and connects the victim and the perpetrator, taking into consideration that the victims sometimes become perpetrators. The book looks into the physical and mental fate of those who are injured in wars. And it pays particular attention to transgenerational trauma – children of victims such as refugees; daughters and sons of the second generation of perpetrators or victims of the Holocaust. The traces of the Shoa are everywhere. Beyond their imprints on individuals, these omnipresent traces shape the Israeli mentality as a whole, and that is traumatic by itself.

In each of the following chapters, I explore the possible ways of expanding the restricted–traumatic mind to a compassionate mind that can recognize the complexity of reality and the interconnectedness between opposite poles. Overall, these chapters demonstrate in different contexts that recognition of complexity is contingent on finding narcissistic balance. It places individual trauma in the context of universal human suffering, which helps the individual gain freedom from post-traumatic loneliness and gain a sense of belonging. Clinical situations and examples illustrate this line of psychoanalytic work and define the role of faith in psychoanalysis.

In Chapter 1, "Captive in a Disaster: October 2023," I introduce the events that took place in the wake of the catastrophic attack on Israel in October 2023 and the war that followed from the perspective of ordinary Israelis who are caught up in the tragedy through family ties, professional involvement, and excessive exposure to distressing images. Two clinical cases, one about a father whose son is being called up to the army and the other about a bereaved mother, illustrate different ways of coping with disaster and restoring vertical splits. Freud's concept of "the uncanny" is used to demonstrate dreadful events as near to experience as possible.

Chapter 2, "Seeing Beyond Blindness," introduces the paradox of knowing and not-knowing. Bion's and Kohut's theoretical contributions are used as a basis for a contextual perspective. I discuss a wide array of transformations of the mind: from emotional blindness, not-knowing, and dogmatic thinking to containing, and knowing, and finally to a transcendental mode of being. Knowing and its evolution to transcendental being signify the ultimate expansion of the mind beyond its cohesive, formative state. A vignette of clinical supervision offered by a leftist therapist to a right-wing patient illustrates the process of transition from the initial state of emotional blindness, archaic narcissism, and hostility to transcendence when compassion becomes possible.

Chapter 3, "Paradoxes of Belonging," presents questions that Israelis are asking themselves: "Where do I really belong?" and "How can I cultivate a broad perspective on contradictory self-states?" These are profound issues for many Israelis. Two vignettes, one of a personal account that depicts my relationship with my father and his homeland, Germany, and the other of a segment from an Israeli film, are presented to illustrate the transformation sought to retrieve a secure experience of belonging. I emphasize the importance of a sense of belonging to an ultimate reality. I explore a spiritual journey, which opens up the path toward compassion and understanding of the complexity of belonging and identity.

Chapter 4, "Perpetrators and Victims," describes a group of German and Israeli analysts who, during 14 annual meetings, explored their personal histories and analytic cases on the background of the Holocaust. The group began with the conventional split between "perpetrators" and "victims." The dynamics in the group process led to the renunciation of preconceived attitudes, transforming traumas from private disasters to shared experiences, and acceptance of an ethical code of responsibility for understanding traumatic and extreme events. I present a vignette that illustrates the process of reclaiming unlived experiences and the freeing of the mind from nameless dread. The discussion emphasizes the attaining of a perspective that facilitates understanding the traumatic experience within a larger context.

Chapter 5, "If You Don't See Me, I Will Show You," explores the vicissitudes of love and their narcissistic derivatives. The wish to be loved derives from narcissistic needs that are often mistaken for sexual desire. I emphasize that therapeutic relations can be conducted in conjunction with gentle love, expressed in a language of tenderness while maintaining the paradox of play and reality. However, when the narcissistic matrix is not sufficiently balanced, and the post-traumatic self is desperate to alleviate its suffering, tender sexuality may give way to sexualization with a perverted inclination. Analysts can disempower these inclinations by maintaining an empathic and compassionate stance. I illustrate these processes with clinical examples.

Chapter 6, "Selfobject Needs as a Mirror of States of the Mind at Times of Environmental Threat and Discontent," relates to unaccustomed challenges at times of social and political upheaval, when a complex external reality affects both patient and analyst, and the walls of the analytic setting collapse. The key question is how to maintain the clinical setup when the analyst and the patient are exposed to a common external threatening reality. Three different patterns of selfobject needs emerge: archaic grandiosity, twinship, and clarity of mind. In this chapter, I point out that patients' reactions to the stressful situation strongly impact the analyst's responses.

The patient's and analyst's responses are entangled and therefore lead to distinctive dialogues in different situations.

Chapter 7, "Accepting Transience,: Relinquishment of the Ego or an Expansion of the Mind?" provides a detailed discussion of the Freudian concept of "transience" and Kohut's elaboration of this concept. In addition to coming to terms with death, Kohut identified the joy and hope that may be inherent in accepting transience. Here, I consider the paradox that transience can be both a disruptive phenomenon and an experience that uncovers the infinite potentiality of self-transformations. I present excerpts from Bionian studies and Buddhist thinking to enrich the investigation. I present an example that illustrates the transformation from defensive attachment to acceptance of transience in the course of therapy.

Chapter 8, "Virtual Reality as a Selfobject Function," illustrates how VR can promote the reclaiming of unlived potentialities, unconscious or disavowed. Using Kohut's concept of the "Virtual Self," I suggest that virtual aspects of the self are unconscious (or unknown) until met by someone or something that encourages their transformation into a conscious state of mind and supports their realization. Two vignettes, drawn from ancient myths, demonstrate how the virtual zone has inspired transformation and expansion of self-awareness from ancient times. A third vignette is presented to illustrate how, with the advent of social media, disavowed and dissociated needs are channeled into cyberspace as communications that are unconsciously geared to reclaim unlived potentialities.

Chapter 9, "Transformation of a Traumatized Mind in Five Dreams," presents five dreams from different stages in the course of a six-year therapy. The dreamer experienced a horrific trauma during his service in the army, in the course of which he was seriously wounded by friendly fire. The dream work promoted a transformation of self-fragmentation to a cohesive self, aware of its destiny and its relation to its environment. This change is apparent in the transference relationship that can be identified in each of the dreams. I discuss a possible link between dreaming and meditation. Both practices consist of imagery, whether it is dreaming or intentional visualization.

Chapter 10, "Emptiness, Equanimity, and the Selfobject Function," draws links between the selfobject function and two major Buddhist concepts: *emptiness* and *equanimity*. The selfobject function and these Buddhist concepts are based on the belief that transformations of the mind are dependent on context. The selfobject function enhances transformations of archaic narcissism to mature narcissism. The Buddhist tradition strives to obtain similar ideals while offering distinctive practices that promote these transformations. In this chapter, I demonstrate how Buddhist thinking contributes to the analytic process.

Chapter 11, "Forms and Transformations of Intergenerational Trauma," uses two Greek myths, Oedipus and Odysseus, to explore patterns of transgenerational trauma. Oedipus illustrates the blind transmission of trauma, which characterizes the experience of many patients whose parents suffered during World War II and subsequently. The hushed background permeated the next generation's psyche. In contrast, Odysseus exemplifies an intergenerational connection in which intersubjectivity, compassion, and empathy are maintained, together with responsibility for caring for peace in the next generation. I present a clinical case that illustrates how, in the course of an analysis, selfobject transferences help patients to become different parents, different persons, who exist creatively in an Odyssean mode.

It is noteworthy that Heinz Kohut, Donald Winnicott, and Alfred Bion – all psychoanalysts of the post-World War II period – are the theoretical cornerstones of this work. They experienced the horrors of World War II and witnessed the impact of historical and cultural contexts on human beings. The psychology that they present is sensitive to human suffering but also to that which is beyond the particular individual. I describe these conceptions alongside more contemporary authors. Buddhist concepts are used to supplement the psychoanalytic line of thought.

Foreword

Tragedy and Transformation: The Contribution of Israeliness to Psychoanalysis

Raanan Kulka

When Heinz Kohut presented his thinking to the psychoanalytic community on human nature's transition from Guilty Man to Tragic Man, few understood the scale of the proposed cultural voyage in terms of both the psychology of ethics and the philosophy of science. Fifty years on, do we recognize the extent of the epistemic, ontological, and ethical changes that arose from this voyage? I dare to suggest that even now, we are a long way from a full understanding of the transcendence that Kohut proposed.

But the revolutionary advance in psychoanalysis concealed in the Kohutian thought is not limited to the transformation from the Guilty Man to the Tragic Man. The contemporary era in self psychology, and even more so in Israeli self psychology, suggests an additional transition – from Tragic Man to Transformed Man. The Transformed Man fully realizes his narcissistic growth and moves from a situation in which the grandiose self is the center of the being that seeks its fulfillment to a space in which the ideal selfhood of being a selfobject guides the destiny of the individual's life. While the Tragic Man lives his personal transformation in the grief of aloneness imposed on him by the splitting of the environment from self, the Transformed Man lives entirely joyfully in a space of total selfobject functioning. Because even in the face of absolute estrangement from the environment that has failed to hold him, he does not split from it, remaining entirely its selfobject with no residue.

The last stanza in the immortal prayer by Shantideva, the 8th-century Buddhist dharma teacher, is an archetypal example of the Transformed Man avoiding dichotomy within himself and toward the world, even in an environment riven by hatred and all-pervasive divisiveness that threatens to drown every trace of the life force in despair and failure: In Shantideva's words "For as long as space endures, and for as long as living beings remain, Until then, may I, too, abide, To dispel the misery of the world."

In all generations, Buddhist texts define the ideal of the Bodhisattva as a "spiritual warrior," as one who achieves an enlightened state of mind that the individual longs for and strives to attain. This state of mind includes a withdrawal from egocentric-solipsistic grandiosity and transcendence to a state of consciousness that seeks to eradicate and heal the sufferings of all those in a state of awareness through the complete commitment to become a selfobject, a spiritual warrior.

The Roots of Spirituality in Israeli Psychoanalysis

The human condition puts man at all times at a junction between self-fulfillment and a commitment to universality, between an individual existence that is true to itself, seeking to achieve self-expression and authenticity, and a supra-individual participation in the world. The supra-individualistic state of mind consists of a commitment to an altruistic state of being, lending a helping hand across the world to every "other" so as to continue, in turn, to engage in the existential choice between self-fulfillment and a commitment to altruism.

The words are boundless because the subject is immeasurable, and all our lives are assembled under its roof. But life's situations, be they big or small, are invariably in the here and now, in our hands at every moment. A tired woman wakes up to the crying of her child in the other room. She gets up and barely pulls herself together; the soles of her feet touch the cold winter floor. But then she withdraws into herself, refusing to respond to appeals, wanting to gather her strength and go back to sleep. Suddenly, she staggers to the bed of her howling infant, who calms down, perhaps merely due to the reassuring sound of her mother's feet, signaling that the woman was prioritizing her child's needs rather than her own.

And the father who jumped to embrace his son while he was falling off a cliff tries in his fantasy to save the son with his wrapping body, ready to die so that his son may live, and a patient, tormented by body and soul, tells me that he needs a shield, an armor because he feels like a slug without a home, faced by an unempathic and alienated world. By some strange stroke of fate, when he leaves the consulting room, utterly focused on himself to the point of total introversion, he walks without seeing what is in front of him, and his foot crushes a slug on the doorstep as if it was waiting for him in a karmic, spellbound test. And he, who does not feel the disaster, leaves only me to painfully and forevermore mourn his fate of both the patient and the slug.

The book presented to us concerns itself with the human being's voyages between the pathways of humanity's pendulum, oscillating between introversion and petition to our fellows, immersed in the trauma of an absence of history and home – a lack that is liable to turn us into the protective shield of selfishness – and, on the other hand, the tragedy of seeking an open heart and transformed mind that liberates itself to reach a fellow being. Yet they realize that their fellow has become an "other," inattentive, unavailable, as if not wanting the gift they have offered him. But Gabriela Mann's book is also concerned with the last stage of narcissistic development, during which a person, filled with joy, discovers the infinity inherent in him, precisely at the very moment when he takes the step of relinquishing himself toward the other.

Thus, this is a book not only written by an esteemed Israeli psychoanalyst endowed with a sensitive heart and the right spirit. It is an Israeli book about Israeli psychoanalysis, a book about the contribution of Israeliness to psychoanalysis. Israel is an admirable cultural–historical rarity in the history of the world's psychoanalytic movement, the full story of which is still waiting to be written. I do not venture to write a strictly accurate historical sketch of that story here but merely to offer a few thoughts by someone who has lived his psychoanalytic life in Israel for more than four decades.

For many years, we resembled a province of a metropolis, nurturing ourselves by the inspiring roots of European psychoanalysis, clinging to the diverse branches of the various disciplines launched by Freud, and onwards to the contributions of his students and colleagues, enthusiastically following historical figures who commenced their journey from Europe to the British Isles and America, both as an organic development and, of course, as a consequence of the great human disasters of the 20th century.

As in every cultural province, we were not merely unique students of the founding fathers and mothers, honoring and acknowledging the sources we relied on, often much more so than others who were more closely associated with them. It was precisely because of our obvious marginality that we secretly became the faithful keepers of the theory and its ethics. Moreover, as citizens of the province, we were not bound by loyalty to any one single figure. In fact, here we were freed from any form of dogmatism, which enabled us to benefit from all the approaches in the psychoanalytic world. That is how, for example, the origin of Israeli psychoanalysis was rooted in both the Freudian and the Jungian perspectives: Max Eitingon and the "guilty man" on the one hand and Erich Neumann and the "mystic man" on the other. Even if the systems of psychoanalytic ideas maintained the political–organizational splits, the psychoanalytic culture that developed here in Israel was typified by a polyvocality that characterizes confluences of varied and diverse currents of thought. It is a juncture at which these ideas fuse and evolve, enriching those who are prepared to open their minds to everyone. We resembled an urban transit community situated between trade and cultural routes heading in every direction, open to the world, familiar with all its languages and ways, even though we were born on the margins of the great events of psychoanalytic history that reached our doorstep.

This was precisely why Israel evolved into a powerful psychoanalytic community, not only in terms of its size but also in relation to all the decisive parameters: the number of female and male analysts in Israel; the total number of psychoanalytic students in a range of formal training programs, both traditional and contemporary; the number of analyses taking place in the country at the same time; and the increasing diversity of the population in analysis, being of every age from kindergarten children to people in the latter years of their lives. All these parameters hold an unrivaled position across the globe, even when compared to the great traditional centers of psychoanalysis.

Therefore, it is not surprising that given this abundance, our position, and the consolidation of our existence, we were able to emerge from being "a hidden recipient" to being openly exposed to the world as a leading psychoanalytic force, both as individuals and as representatives of the community, participating not only as passive recipients of knowledge but also as active contributors, beginning to present its own scientific community to the wider world with unique and unknown contours which stimulate curiosity and interest. However, at the same time, we were still students of the teachers we visited in the world (or those we invited here for a brief stay or for years). By this time, we were already becoming recognized and gaining amity and appreciation while still retaining the status of students.

The writing of a book by a person whose collective works form a corpus of thought and practice indicates a powerful change of mind that transforms a person from a student to a teacher. This is the change that, even if its humble beginnings already emerged during our era as a province about two decades ago by pioneers who dared to spread their wings, there is now a clear sign of the maturation of the psychoanalytic scene in Israel, which is increasingly distinguished by more and more original Israeli works in psychoanalysis. Gabriela Mann's book, which is now making its way into the public mind, brings with it a novel uniqueness in that it not only is an original personal work on psychoanalysis but also tells the story of the evolution of a unique psychoanalysis that is conceived and researched in Israel.

On Consciousness and the Mind

Practicing Psychoanalysis in Israel: Seeing Through Blindness is the concise title of Gabriela Mann's book. A profound challenge to conventional psychoanalysis is concealed behind the modesty of the title, which transfers us, seemingly unintentionally, from the realms of the conscious to the space of the mind. The humane language that signifies the world is embarrassed to contain the spiritual dimensions of humanity and express them. However, the linguistic leap from the word consciousness to the word mind embodies the basic premise of the book, according to which the mind is not just limited to consciousness, the realm within which there is a representation of the constant link between us and the world and everything in it. The word mind clearly signals the transition from the epistemic as the objective of psychoanalysis – the expansion of consciousness that knows itself – to the expansion of consciousness that offers itself to the world as psychoanalysis's objective of an existential human aspiration. This signals a transition to the ontological and, even more so, to the ethical.

It is not our role here and now to set sail into the expanses of generations of human philosophy with regard to the fundamental questions about the human psyche and spirit. The book's title invites us to what is already contained in it, the developing relationship between psychoanalysis and Buddhism, a relationship that the author spreads out with moderate but determined gentleness throughout every section of the book, at times implicitly and at other times by way of a focused observation. The English word "mind" was chosen as her translation of the word "chitta," which in Sanskrit means consciousness and in translation lends itself to several words in Hebrew. In the context of this book, I choose the word "spirit," which usually occurs in the space between the two common words "consciousness" and "mind."

In psychoanalytic discourse, for reasons of communicative convenience, we tend to give up the subtle differences between the two words. But the psychological thought of Buddhism distinguishes between consciousness, which carries the dual structure of body–mind, which is a phenomenon that goes beyond any duality, a kind of space where all phenomena emerge and into which they dissolve. The human mind is a sixth sense, not a system of processing the impressions of the five senses. Buddhist metaphysics and psychology engage the sixth sense as an event all of its own, located beyond the stored and functioning contents of the psyche. It therefore completely transcends any mental dynamics. Even if I am guilty of overgeneralization, it can be said in the present context that while the expansion of consciousness is related to the expansion of the boundaries of the human psyche, the expansion of the mind is the expansion of the dimensions of man's transformation, the widening of his retreat from the distinct personal self, toward his cosmic selfhood, which is the full surrender inherent in us, which in Buddhist teachings, is understood as reaching the realm of enlightenment.

On the first page of his book, *The Analysis of the Self*, Kohut (1971) mentions that the objective of analysis is to reach inner peace and happiness. It is difficult to think of a more decisive watershed when discussing the difference between the stage of the foundation of psychoanalysis, as suggested to human civilization by Freud, and the revolutionary act that Kohut contemplates for the future evolution of the discipline. Freud was wary of the words "peace and happiness" and of the infrastructure of a dialectical struggle between life and death, which imposes on us a constant cycle of inherent restlessness and constant suffering. Freud's caution in using these terms was, from his perspective, a guideline to his understanding of the world and its inhabitants. Kohut, however, offers a very different prospect: inner peace and happiness.

Kohut's courageous approach, which prevails in Gabriela Mann's book, derives from the fact that the basic human condition of empathy, which defines the very dimension of psychology in the world, is fundamentally the reverse of the Freudian premise in relation to the ontological split that exists between one person and another and therefore also within each and every person. The non-dual worldview confronts us with the claim that there is no self without a selfobject. The very assumption of total oneness that exists in the entire world of phenomena presumes that the inner nature of the human spirit is not one of splitting and separation but rather a state of peaceful wholeness characterized by happiness. Therefore, there is no reason to wonder that for Kohut, accepting the feasibility of inner peace and happiness is not one of human hubris, which necessitates the maturation of a submissive acceptance of man's limitations. For if man is separated from the world, then the premise of constant restlessness and suffering is correct, but if the basic assumption is unity, the postulation of peace and happiness is a rational derivative.

"Know thyself" was the maxim inscribed on the wall of the ancient temple in Delphi. This dictum was adopted by psychoanalysis to suggest man's objective in life. It came to be an imperative marking of the transition from unconscious to consciousness, a saying that may be the source of the definition of psychoanalysis as Depth Psychology, matters hidden from recognition which have not yet become known and which need to be known so that an individual can be a wise and complete person. The psychoanalytic psychology known as Spacial self psychology demands that the maxim "Know your neighbor" be imprinted on our minds and – perhaps even more so – "Be to your neighbor" (Kulka, 2010).

The conceptual movement embodied in the transition from Depth Psychology to a Psychology of Space can be achieved by placing two additional elements to Descartes's immortal saying, "I think therefore I am" and "I exist therefore I exist." This is a maxim of existentialism that sanctifies existence and frees man from the burden of confirming his experience with wisdom intelligence. The current element, presented to us by self psychology and the psychology of selfobjecting, is the unique product of an Israeli creation. It is clearly conveyed in this book, in the sense of "I realize, therefore I exist."

The psychological transformation from my investment in myself to my profound immersion in my other is anchored in the narcissistic–spiritual development of the individual, who can let go of his self-grasping and move to a position of compassionate empathy and valuing the other. It is this movement of transformation that liberates an individual from his existential suffering and opens for him a space of tranquility and happiness. This position of human nature and its growth are shared by two conceptions that are entangled in the book – self psychology and the Buddhist dharma.

Gabriela Mann's book demonstrates the way in which these two concepts are repeatedly interwoven and evolve. Already at the beginning of the book, the author lays the foundation for the moving ideas that the reader will encounter throughout it and declares that blindness is inherent in the hermetic attachment to ourselves. It is the source of our suffering.

Buddhist dharma uses the term "ignorance" to describe our attachment to ourselves. It is the cause of a diminishing mind and human suffering. Only the liberation of the mind can ensure the dissolution of suffering, the evacuation of its roots, and their purification.

The figure of the blind man in psychoanalysis alternates between Tiresias and Oedipus, between the prophet who sees with the eyes of his mind and the man who refuses to know the innermost parts of his being. When the tragedy reaches its climax, Oedipus's ignorant blindness, the blindness bound by his repressed fate, is replaced by the blindness of the body that Oedipus inflicts on himself as a punishment for the guilt surging within him as the truth is revealed. But doesn't the blindness of the body bring him to the realms of prophecy, to the dominion of the spirit, which releases him from being the Guilty Man to becoming the Tragic Man? We will, in due course, return to Oedipus's mythological status in psychoanalysis' inheritance and the obstacle it poses to its next stage of development.

Trauma and Tragedy

When the word psychoanalysis appeared for the first time in 1896 (Freud, 1962), it marked the decisive transition between the seduction theory as the basis of the explanation for the hysterical mental disorder and the paradigmatic breakthrough in the discovery of the unconscious as a basis for the coming into being of the neurotic disorder. Although this was a seminal moment for the inimitable discipline of Depth Psychology, it distanced psychoanalysis from understanding the trauma that comes from mortal harm to human beings by the forces of nature, catastrophic events, and the terrible actions of humans toward each other, alongside the emergence of an exciting scientific paradigm, which offered an understanding of the unconscious layers of the mind and the coming into being of fantasies that distort the individual's perception of reality. Psychoanalysis failed to continue to be a source of inspiration and relief for the understanding of realistic trauma and its destabilizing impact to the point of total undermining of the human psyche.

It is no wonder that revolutionary cultural and social factors that surfaced at the beginning of the 20th century and continue to the present day, from Marxism to Feminism, disowned psychoanalysis with the painful accusation aimed at all its admirers' claims that it ignores the external reality and its effects on an individual's mind and his fate. It took many decades for psychoanalysis to re-represent itself to human society, illustrate its relevance to the question of trauma in human life, and propose theoretical paradigms that deal not only with the unconscious processes of the mind but also with the essence of man's being and his existential situation within the natural, social, economic, and political environment in which he lives out his life. The rescue of psychoanalysis from being merely a subordinate of the intrapsychic and reaching the understanding that it must dare to also be a complete contextual theory of the interpersonal and the historical restored it to its novel status as a total psychology that is a worthy foundation for anyone who seeks to protect the human and humanity.

The realization that trauma is not merely a distinct, defined, one-off, acute event but was also the harbinger of sprawling processes that lead to secondary malignant metastasizing growths occurred after the world wars. Thus, postwar psychoanalysis, faced with horrific ongoing psychological disorders of varying forms and content, began to seek a metatheoretic understanding that would interweave intrapsychic processes – the objects of classical psychoanalytic research – with external environmental processes, which initiate a novel psychoanalytic perspective.

Self psychology had a unique role to play in this process, which, in a surprising and revolutionary way, led it back into the arms of classical psychology. This was due to its definition of a traumatic event as a pure psychic event without splitting it from the experience that determines consciousness. While the definition of trauma with all its theoretical–clinical innovations remained linked to an unusual event that does not stem from the individual human being, external to the event, "external" in this context is perceived as separate from the individual's experiencing of the trauma. Self psychology assumes that the trauma originates from failures in the proper functioning of the basic selfobject psychological matrix. Although from an external perspective, the selfobject link ostensibly occurs between two – the self and his selfobject – this is not an interactive relationship between two entities intrinsic to themselves and separate from each other but an event of a dimension of a revolutionary nature in the history of the philosophy of science; it is an occurrence of non-dual interbeing, in which the selfobject is the self external to himself not a subject in its own right. The self is, therefore, in a kind of affinity with itself that is neither an intrapsychic nor an interpersonal existence but rather an event that meets spiritual quantum definitions of a supra-individual occurrence.

The elimination of the division between inner and outer, inherent in the radical conceptualization of the selfobject function, discounts the definition of trauma from the duality that afflicted psychoanalysis in its painful relationship with the question of human trauma. In this way, self psychology responds both to the sensitivity of the present era of humanity, which is seeking its ethical development against any wrongdoing or disaster, and to the renewal of the view of trauma as a purely psychological event.

In one of his many inspiring statements, Kohut (1985b) suggests that while classical psychoanalysis reveals the sorrow of the child in the adult and identifies the failures of the past in the emergence of a normal and healthy present, self psychology brings to light the sadness of the adult in the child and so locates the failures of the present in relation to the evolution of an appropriate and brimming future. The self always possesses the potential for future realization. At each and every moment of the present, it is in need of a formative link to the empathic functions of the selfobject.

In other words, the self is always a virtual self that is not yet realized and awaits its inception by an empathic sustaining matrix. In the absence of such a matrix, the self of the "now moment" will not evolve into its future, which constitutes the ultimate definition of trauma. Therefore, according to self psychology, trauma occurs from one moment to another, and it does not require extraordinary or irregular events in either their nature or their intensity from what is considered the "norm." Human existence within the narcissistic system constitutes man constantly vulnerable to situations of insufficient and unstable empathic nurturing. It thus turns man's vulnerability into one of the fundamental signs of his being. The "normality" of the trauma intrinsic to this perception takes the ethical dimension in psychoanalysis to its peak in that it conditions the person's situation as being dependent on the essentiality of total empathy for his immediate surroundings.

At this point, I would like to suggest that the inclusive manner in which self psychology perceives trauma transforms it into a fundamental definition of human tragedy and, in so doing, clarifies an additional layer to the conceptualization of the Tragic Man suggested by Kohut to psychoanalysis and human culture. Gabriela Mann places the transition from traumatic to tragic as being an emerging focal point of her book, and its chapters, with their metatheoretical propositions and the human-clinical examples interwoven in each of them, create a particularly rich mosaic of indications, how we can detect tragic dimension in trauma's ubiquitous presence. The tragedy is fully exposed when an expansive perspective reveals that the trauma spreading throughout the world has no beginning and no end and that it eradicates the linear duality between victimizer and victim and entirely invalidates the question: "Who started it?" This question is implied without any hesitation in relation to responsibility; at any given moment, there is a definite ethical and tangible responsibility that cannot be differentiated between the abuser and the abused, between an offender and his victim.

But a psychoanalytic examination will always endlessly expand the perspective of the unique trauma and reveal the diverging paths of the contextual tapestry of suffering that has no beginning and no end. This is exactly how the full investigation of the Oedipus myth will reveal that the murder of the father and the incestuous relationship with the mother began with the attempted murder by Laius and Jocasta of their son Oedipus. And even this catastrophic crime did not begin purposelessly as an expression of the death instinct that unfolds in hatred and aggression from which there is no escape but has further roots in the curse conferred on Laius, according to which any son born to him would murder him in retribution for his original crime of kidnapping and possibly sexually abusing the son of King Pelops, who had sheltered him from his enemies. And, of course, these mythological connections go further and further back in history ad infinitum.

The psychoanalytic perspective suggested by Gabriela Mann's book does not absolve any of us from responsibility. It does, however, attempt to extract us from the experience of being the Guilty Man and Tragic Man due to the universal cognizance of trauma and the understanding that a trauma inflicted upon me could, with ease, unconsciously find its place in my inner being, leading to viewing it as the cause of the trauma that I myself will, in turn, wreak upon my surroundings. Therefore, the most destructive impact of any trauma is related to the ethical stance of the human spirit. Known mechanisms of projection and projective identification are liable to create a limitless tragic chain of traumas that never end.

Was Cain guilty of murdering Abel? He certainly was. And for that he was duly punished. However, the punishment was accompanied by God's attempt to prevent the next murder by the holy mark imprinted on the forehead of the first person who took the life of another, lest anyone think that Cain's act of murder was permissible, thereby making the next murder acceptable. Did the murder of Abel originate the deed of murdering? Of course not. God stimulated the split between the first human beings, Cain and Abel. Jealousy and competition, hatred and rage, are the agents of this dissension between us; they are not its psychological origin but only the channels through which the blind, failed idea of separateness flows cruelly. Cain and Abel are the paradigmatic symbols of the Guilty Man and the Tragic Man that we all are. However, they have the capacity to transcend those symbols by becoming the spiritual man, the one who contributes to the dissolution of the separateness, which causes the trauma present in everything.

In the chapters of her book, Gabriela Mann submits the idea of an evolutionary movement between three stages that are both theoretical and clinical: (1) validating the individual's particular traumatic experience, which facilitates the recovery of his pre-traumatic potential self; (2) accommodating the universality of trauma in human life, so enabling an individual to be freed from post-traumatic loneliness and to regain a sense of human belonging; and (3) the transformation of the human mind from an egocentric attachment that is blind to the totality of the link between human beings; a spiritual position that constantly and selflessly seeks to attain an altruistic position toward the other and in so doing promotes the realization of the joy of the spiritual man.

The author is able to extract the "area of faith," to use Michael Eigen's (1981) inspirational term, from psychoanalytic history and its collective works. The concept brings together reflections, ideas, and concepts collated from various paradigmatic schools in the history of psychoanalysis and woven into a fascinating thesis. Winnicott, Bion, and Kohut are undoubtedly the cornerstones of such a perspective, alongside contributions from the works of other analysts. However, the main contribution offered by Gabriela Mann's book is the natural way in which she has succeeded in integrating the basic concepts of Buddhist wisdom into psychoanalytic thinking and illustrating this in her therapeutic action. If, in the opening pages of the book, ignorance is viewed as the source of our existential–psychological suffering, the author moves on to rely on love, compassion, joy, and equanimity, the four seats of supreme mindfulness, which guide her thinking and analytic action, on a pathway that frees one from suffering.

The initial release from suffering originates from the transformation processes that the analytical therapist has to go through in her own mind. The book does not directly provide us with a description of the processes of Buddhist study and practice, which the therapist herself undergoes under the guidance of teachers and within a practicing community. However, the author's ability to frankly share clinical experiences that transcend conventional questions of countertransference unveils her parents' life story, that of her family, as well as her own life. Also, it informs us of her political, social, and ethical positions, so forming an illustration of her complete worldview in terms of both human and world issues. Will the processes of mind transformation also be the lot of the patient and not only of the therapist? This question is presented in the most honest and direct way in several chapters of the book, and the question of whether the self can free itself from the embrace of its traumas and sense the deviation from the ego to an expansion of self is presented as a challenging and thorough investigation.

Kohut suggested two distinct ethical positions regarding the processes of transformation, which he believed are the peak of human development. The first position determines that it is entirely legitimate for an individual to remain in the coterie of the narcissistic grandiosity of the self and strive to achieve his ambitions of greatness. In doing so, Kohut was offering humanity the restoration of the dignity of narcissism and its liberation from our judgmental attitude toward it; he completed Freud's initial historical–cultural move of freeing sexuality and aggression from the judgmental position that humankind had adopted in relation to these human phenomena.

The second ethical position suggested by Kohut states that a person's narcissistic development cannot be said to have been completed other than by transformation of mind, leading to a deviation from the self of greatness to an ideal self, leading to a supra-individual existence. Can a person reach such a revolutionary developmental achievement during his lifetime? And, even more so, with the help of psychoanalytic treatment? In the overall corpus of his thought, we find Kohut oscillating on the one hand between the feeling that this achievement is the preserve of only a few of us and, therefore, should not be used as a criterion for the success of the treatment or for evaluating the completeness of a person's life. At the same time, Kohut holds on to the fundamental belief that such a transformation of mind is completely within the scope of what is possible for every person and that analytical treatment is an ideal platform for achieving such an ultimate developmental space.

The freeing of the human collective and the single person from the dual judgmental attitude of the drive and narcissism is one of the decisive achievements of psychoanalysis as a selfobject of history and culture. Its influence on us as human beings and on our civilization is incalculable. But the responsibility of that discipline does not end there: precisely because of the liberation of man embodied in psychoanalysis, it is also the discipline's full responsibility to mold humanity in the period following its liberation from this instinctive and narcissistic tendencies. Its challenge is to deal with two objectives: (1) to prevent the liberation of sexuality from degenerating into a perversion of intimacy and into violation of the sanctity of the human body; and (2) to prevent narcissistic liberation from degenerating into egocentricity, which seeks to subvert the foundations of human unity and, like a fire, destroy the universal dimensions of existence.

Gabriela Mann's faith is tangential to Kohut's. With deep love and compassion, and even with visible inner joy, she accepts the emergence of her patients' wishes for self-fulfillment, even when they are clearly different from her own choices as a person, as a woman, as a psychoanalyst, and as an Israeli, and even completely contradict them. But her total empathy for the grandiose self of her patients does not diminish an iota from positioning herself as an ideal selfobject for the sake of her patients' transformational processes, be they new venues of motherhood, freed from egocentric attachment to children or the space of professional therapists who seek to deepen their total empathy, including toward patients who differ or oppose them in terms of worldviews, or even for those who belong to an adversarial group that caused severe trauma to the therapists, members of their family, and their nation. The consistent commitment to helping people realize and fulfill both poles of their self, the grandiose and the ideal, is the foundation of the author's belief that people can sustain their human recovery from the traumatic wounds inherent in human existence and reach full narcissistic development, both in fulfilling the self's particular ambitions and in the realization of the ideal goals of the universal selfhood.

A philosophical–linguistic pause concerning the words *fulfillment* and *realization* is required here. The place of Israeli self psychology in the assimilation of psychoanalytic concepts in the Hebrew language is an organic part of the development of the Israeli psychoanalytic school of thought. Interlacing psychoanalytic and Buddhist systems of thought contributes additional layers to the formation of an innovative psychology, of which Gabriela Mann's book is an echo. One of the conceptual–linguistic innovations concerns the distinction between fulfillment and realization, words that we usually do not use sufficiently as subtly and sophisticatedly as we do with other words whose meaning is identical. Relying on the dharma, Buddhist wisdom allows us a much higher conceptual resolution; fulfillment is the mode of operation of the untransformed mind, attached to a dualistic perception of the relative reality, and assumes the existence of an intrinsic and separate self. Fulfillment, therefore, accurately describes the mode of operation of the grandiose self with ambitions seeking to be realized, and the so well-known combination of self-fulfillment reflects the philosophical underpinning of the term fulfillment.

On the other hand, realization is the definition of an awakened mind that reaches a full understanding of the absolute reality in which all phenomena are empty of self-existence. Realization therefore accurately describes the longing and striving of the ideal self for the complete transcendental transformation from the egocentric self to the cosmic self. Conceivably, the no less familiar concept of self-transcendence reflects the philosophical underpinning of the term realization. The Buddhist language terms fulfillment "this shore" and realization "the shore opposite." The transition from one bank to the other is regarded as liberation from suffering. And the one who gives his life and his mind and helps others, any other, to cross from one bank to the other, is the one who lives as an "awake being" – a Bodhisattva.

The psychoanalytic area of faith does not consist of human innocence but is the fruit of wisdom, the highest form of transformation. The journey from ignorance to wisdom completes the course of compassion. Like a bird that cannot realize its inner nature of flight except by virtue of its two wings, so too, the complete journey of consciousness from tragedy to transformation requires ultimate narcissistic development and wisdom. The profound contemplative link between the five transformations from self to selfhood, presented to us by Kohut, and the six perfections in Buddhist spirituality inspire wonderment and gratitude. The climax of this amazement is reached via the absolute identity of regarding wisdom as the supreme achievement of cosmic narcissism, in the language of the psychoanalyst or in the language of the Buddhist dharma, "the bank that is beyond."

The philosophical definition of wisdom, be it anchored in the ancient and vast cultural treasure of Buddhism or rediscovered in the course of the last century in the modest but revolutionary cultural treasure of psychoanalysis, is the revelation of the mind that all phenomena are empty of intrinsic existence, transient, and consist of infinite links to other phenomena; all of them are dependent on the mind that constitutes them and supplies them with meaning.

The range of the therapeutic work described in Gabriela Mann's book rapidly reveals a constant movement from compassion to wisdom. So much so that it is almost possible to reach the conclusion that we have been presented with an orderly method of psychoanalytic treatment that begins with the compassionate validation of subjective experience and moves meticulously to reach the realms of wisdom that liberate the individual from himself. This movement undoubtedly echoes one of the inspirational processes in psychoanalysis, which leads from the liberation from the object to liberation from the self. This process invites us to join this spiritual path, where transformative processes formulated in self psychology are interwoven with Buddhist formulations with regard to the steps that lead to the awakening of the mind.

The 13th-century Zen Master Dōgen encapsulated the process of being exposed to us with the wisdom of an enlightened mind: to learn the Buddha's truth is to learn ourselves, to learn ourselves is to forget ourselves, to forget ourselves is to be experienced by the myriad dharmas.

The Israeli Tragedy

The existential coordinates of the Israeli being that I wish to establish in this essay extend between two axes. The first, the Shoah, is the traumatic infrastructure of Israeli existence, a trauma that throbs within us as both a historical and an ethical justification. The second is the national identity of Israel's existence as a distinct entity unto itself. These two axes are, enigmatically and unexpectedly, inseparably entangled with each other. Rather than diminishing and weakening with the passage of time, they, in fact, become increasingly entrenched in the individual psyche of the majority and in the collective spirit that defines us.

Modesty prevents me from offering here an orderly subtext for these deep processes. Their cultural, social, and political deciphering naturally colonizes everything that exists and has happened in this special place over the course of the last three generations. I do, however, wish to depict at least a small part of the modest contribution of psychoanalysis to the understanding and explanation of the Israeli tragedy. The psychoanalytic contribution to the mosaic of conceptual and historical thought about Israeliness is still in its infancy. Unfortunately, it seems that the psychoanalytic community in Israel tends to largely avoid adopting a determined stance that would offer the outcome of its work in this field to both the general and the professional Israeli public. This apprehension relates to the possible arrogant misuse of disciplinary expertise in the dialogue between worldviews and the justified fear of diluting a scientific discipline by dabbling in tangible questions of everyday life. However, one must never allow the arguments that nurture the natural anxiety about the politicization of a scientific discipline to serve as the rationale, albeit the easiest, for the idea of "the treason of the psychoanalysts."

When, in 1927, Julien Benda (2006) coined the astonishing and highly inspiring term "the betrayal of intellectuals," his complex cogitation contained two major principles that define the experience of the intellectual. These principles remained somewhat concealed and prevented a complete understanding of the depth of Benda's term. The first is the phenomenological nature of man, which is revealed in innumerable disastrous acts of injustice that he perpetrates on others and on the world and does not reflect the inner core of his character. Consequently, Benda leaves utopia intact, not as a denial of reality or as an irrational illusion but as a possibility that man may return to his true nature, his good nature. Relying on the Shoah as one of the pillars of Israeliness is an unconscious collective reflection of the acceptance of the death instinct as the basic principle of life, which reinforces trauma as a permanent feature of the solitary and social person. The Shoah therefore shapes the mental-spiritual existence of Israeliness as an unchangeable occurrence of tragedies that distances the Israeli existence from the potentially beneficial reliance on utopia.

The second principle inherent in Julien Benda's concept concerns the complex issue that exists between the particular concrete and the universal principle. While the sanctification of the particular within the visible relative reality distances and disconnects us from the unifying and universal in our being, the absolute reality, defined by universality, holds in its lap the particular without any duality. The constant strengthening of the Israeli national identity, while increasingly dissociated from every inclusive aspect of human universality, leaves Israeliness in the sphere of an experience of loneliness and lack of belonging. The blind trust in self-sufficiency disregards the recognition of the profundity in the inherent interconnectedness of all that exists in the universe. This blinded ignorance leads to an experience of discontent, dissatisfaction, and existential suffering that define the Israeli tragedy.

By echoing diverse cultural reflections across generations of human civilization, Banda suggests that the intellectual, the person of spirit, is the one who does not only **live** the life of what exists at any given moment but also reflects on what there is. In Banda's view, the person who contemplates what exists is the one who, on behalf of us all and the universal good, holds on to the utopian ideal. This spiritual assumption determines that since there is no person who does not reflect on existence and existing, then every person is an intellectual. The problem is that alongside the position that regards every person of awareness as a spiritual entity that simultaneously holds the universal and the utopian, we know, as do others, how great the temptation is to abandon the reflective position, to defeat ourselves and betray our deeper nature.

"Sciences of reflection" – contemplative sciences – are today viewed as all those spiritual sciences that are concerned with the inner nature of those who have a mind. Over a long period of time, I have suggested that we define the science of psychoanalysis as the last of the sciences of reflection that man has sought to create in the cultural world (Kulka, 2019). This turns the psychoanalytic thoughts and actions into an act that takes place between intellectuals, regardless of their cultural–educational biographical background. Is there a more appropriate space than psychoanalysis, where the utopian potential of the unity of the particular and the universal is manifested in its highest form?

Gabriela Mann's book is a living testimony to the possibility – accessible to all of us – not to betray the "treason of those who contemplate." It clearly demonstrates the contribution of psychoanalysis to the political sphere in the broadest sense of the word. Gabriela Mann is a courageous model of the ethical stability of a psychoanalyst who is not afraid to realize the unique potential of the psychoanalytic position as a place from which we can be selfobjects, validating the particular subjectivity of the individual and at the same time initiate a transformative universal spirit. Throughout the various chapters of the book, the theoretical and clinical processes lead from the individual to the supra-individual, from the subject with the unique identity entitled to his singular voice to the individual who chooses to transform and recognize his privilege to be an entire selfobject to each other. In one of Kohut's immortal statements, he suggests that "every case of psychopathology is not only an individual maladjustment but also an example of an attempt to find a new solution to man's psychological problems" (Kohut, 1985a). In so doing, Kohut establishes the theoretical and tangible infrastructure for a non-dual amalgam of the grandiose self who is extricated from his suffering through a transformation into the ideal selfhood that longs for and strives to solve human problems.

The beginning of the Israeli tragedy is reflected in the vicissitudes of fate presented in the different treatments, including the treatment of those whose fate it was to be among the victims of World War II, those murdered, their murderers, refugees, and the daughters and sons of the second and third generations of perpetrators and victims. But the chronic continuation of our tragedies is not in the trauma of the Shoah, which is beyond representation, including the struggle in regard to forgetting and remembering. The Shoah will accompany humanity forever. The continuation of the tragedy emanates from the processes of projective identification, which threatens through its warped and twisted sophisticated prism to turn the oppressed into oppressors.

The justified need and necessity to recognize the pain resulting from the horrors of that war soon becomes the reasoning for our alienation from the other whom we disavow and seemingly cleanly define as "other." From that point on, we find ourselves close to being able to heartlessly justify the pain we cause, the dimensions of which may grow due to the vertical split within which we live and which allows us to completely abandon the ability to naturally convert to empathy. Abandoning empathy and other zones of transformation, such as love, compassion, joy, and courage, resembles a betrayal of ourselves, which we can hardly perceive due to the depletion of our mind and spirit up to dehumanization of our own selfhood. Yet, that is not the end of the horrible process of the incarnations of projective identification that may become a retreat into a black hole of archaic narcissism, which indiscriminately excludes from me anyone who is not me. Soon everyone else becomes "not me," even those who only yesterday were my friends, partners in my group, to which I swore my allegiance and which included my brother, my own flesh and blood, my sister, dear to me as my life. And from there, the realms of perversion, violent psychopathy, and insanity break loose without any reservations.

The occupation and settlement, the First Lebanon War and Rabin's assassination, the evacuation of the Gaza Strip settlements and the Second Lebanon War. Blood and fire and billows of smoke, endless circles of suffering and disaster, disputes of hatred and splits of rage colonize the history of our lives and the lives of all the others who are with us and around us and are visible to us as the heroes of this book, Gabriela Mann's patients. Ami, one of the protagonists, the patient who was injured by friendly fire while serving in the reserves, is himself an expression of the peak that gradually evolves throughout the book, a kind of collectively binding story that embodies the state of collapse in which we already find ourselves. It is a phase of self-harm, of directing death toward ourselves, of the final abandonment of our humanity. The circle of Israeli tragedies seems to complete its winding journey from the vital confrontation with the enormity of the trauma of the Shoah as its clear victims through to the proven danger awaiting us of harming others. And finally, we reach a psychological solidarity in which we directly harm ourselves, a kind of existence in absolute solitude in the absence of all "others."

The Contribution of Israeliness to Psychoanalysis

Can we overcome the Israeli tragedy? Can we once again reverse the direction of the movement of the wheel and rid ourselves of the toxic collective projective identification in which we live? The decisive contribution of the psychoanalytic essay that is presented to us lies in the full belief that the psychoanalysis of the expansion of the mind and the psychoanalysis of transformation have a positive answer to these fateful questions about the future of Israeliness, perhaps even about the very future of Israel.

The courage needed to cut the Gordian knot between the wronged and the righteous in an infinite circular chain of tragedy resembles the courage that requires psychoanalysis to abandon the Oedipus myth and join each other by agreeing to adopt the myth of Odysseus. Oedipus will never be able to rescue humanity, neither from egocentric blindness and hubris nor from the endless struggles between fathers and sons, sons and fathers. Therefore, Oedipus will always reflect the misery of binding, the original binding, having his ankles bound with a long sewing pin by his parents, Laius and Jocasta, who left him to die in the wilderness on Mount Kithairon. So it will be for all the others who follow, like Ami, who was killed by friendly fire. As in Orwell's shameful expression that makes us all both victimizers and victims in a terrifying vicious circle.

Odysseus, whom Kohut calls the first war refuser because of his desire to be a spouse and a devoted father to his wife and son, is the one who believes in a fundamental alliance between the generations, a faith that leads him to solidarity, compassion, and altruism, which are based on the withdrawal from the idea of separateness that divides as the explanation of man. And perhaps Odysseus's refusal to go to war was not just an evasion to remain in the bosom of his family but a much deeper ethical statement, this one against the idea of the self in itself and for itself?

Kohut's last paper, "Introspection, Empathy, and the Semi-Circle of Mental Health" (1982), was written as a lecture in honor of the fiftieth anniversary of the Chicago Psychoanalytic Institute. Kohut no longer had the privilege of presenting it himself to his colleagues, and its delivery was entrusted to his son, Thomas Kohut, who read the paper at the jubilee ceremony. In this farewell essay, Kohut offers psychoanalysis the character of Odysseus as someone who made the journey from grandiosity to ideals, from emergence to dissolution, and from form to transformation. The transformation is what ends Odysseus's tormenting journeys. This is why he deserves to be a mythical human hero who paves the way for us, psychoanalysts, toward rescuing man from endless trauma and tragedies.

Israeli self psychology has embraced the myth of Odysseus with all its heart, and in its avant-garde moves in the last decade, it is indeed striving for the distillation of a psychoanalysis of presence based on a metatheory of the transformation of the mind. "The tragedy of my life is that my parents don't know anything about me," says Betty, one of Gabriela Mann's analysands, when she gathers around the analyst's empathic presence and begins, perhaps for the first time in her life, to feel that there is someone in the world who recognizes her life. From this point on, the flow of the woman's life changes, the daughter of parents burdened with historical and personal traumas who are immersed in the wounds of their narcissism, while she is psychologically abandoned, hollow, and lost. Her return to her pre-traumatic self, as the author's original conception, opens up to her the horizon of transformation from which her creativity flows again as a writer who struggled for years with difficult writing inhibitions, as well as a new empathic motherhood is born in her for her daughter. This can be viewed as an Odyssean motherhood that has replaced an Oedipal motherhood, as her analyst would say.

Perhaps it is precisely the one who has experienced a continuous trauma that turns him into the Tragic Man, who must offer himself as the one on whose doorstep there is an invitation to bring about recovery. And this not only for his own sake and that of his relatives and associates but perhaps also for the recovery of those who are supposedly not close to him, all human beings. The Israeli tragedy can be the entity that may also lead to a turning point in the transformation of the mind, which will turn us into a resource of functioning selfobjects of great change, of reparation. The place of Israeli psychoanalysis in such a process is a great prerogative that we should not miss. At the beginning of the discussion, Israel's unique dimension on the global map of psychoanalysis was already emphasized. Toward the end, I would like to suggest that the special work of Israeli self psychology in the interweaving of psychoanalysis with the philosophy and psychology of Buddhism is one of the most inviting expressions of Israeli psychoanalysis for the expansion of the mind and the transformation of the human spirit.

In the winter of 1929, the poet Rachel Bluwstein wrote the words of the poem, which is engraved on her tomb on the shores of the Sea of Galilee.

"From Mount Nevo"

The air listens,
And the heart,
Has he come? Will he come?

In every waiting for,
a never,
The sadness of Nevo.

Shore and shore
Of a single stream
Facing each other.

The stone decree
Apart
Forever
Stretch out a hand
In vain.

There!
No coming to,
A man and his Nevo
On a wide plain.
– Rachel Bluwstein (1929)

How sorrowful and lifting are these lines of wonder? How lucid and refined is the transition from the individual pain of an unrealized meeting of human love to the realms of the universal spirit from which, the poet reminds us, we are all "Moses"? And not only in the simple meaning of the word because, like him, we will also see the land from the other side, and we will not reach it. This, perhaps, is a punishment for an original sin in front of a grumpy Oedipal father. However, we are all endowed with an Odyssean mind, which, in its inner nature, can be a transformed mind of prophecy. It is not for nothing that Moses's burial place is unknown because it is not an earthly fulfillment embodied in the Transfigured Man but rather the realization of a spirit.

The Transformed Man, who lives his life to the fullest extent with courage and joy, is the horizon of the other bank, the shore on the other side. That is not to suggest that it does not exist. Rather, it is an expression of a desire that is not in the sense of something we can yearn for and strive toward or even reach.

In dharma, the teachings of the Buddha, the fourth stage of the spiritual path is called "joyous effort," which represents the moment when the human mind crosses the river, from the shore of ordinary existence, full of suffering and tragedies, to the safe shore of Nevo, and the mind expands and opens a horizon for enlightenment.

Merging into Rachel's inspiration is not a nostalgic embrace of the Israeliness of the past but the deep knowledge that the Israeliness of today, and of every moment, contains within it the natural ability for us, as individuals and as a unique collective, to live ourselves – to forget ourselves – to be at one with everything (Kohut, 1984).

References

Benda, J. (2006). *The treason of the intellectuals* (R. Aldington, Trans.). Routledge (Original work published in 1927).

Freud, S. (1962). Heredity and the aetiology of the neuroses. In *The standard edition of the complete psychological works of Sigmund Freud: Vol. 3 (1893–1899): Early psycho-analytic publications* (pp. 141–156). Hogarth Press.

Kohut, H. (1971). *The analysis of the self: A systematic approach to the psychoanalytic treatment of narcissistic personality disorders*. International Universities Press.

Kohut, H. (1982). Introspection, empathy, and the semi-circle of mental health. *The International Journal of Psycho-Analysis*, *63*(4), 395–407.

Kohut, H. (1984). *How does analysis cure?* (A. Goldberg & P. Stepansky, Eds.). University of Chicago Press.

Kohut, H. (1985a). On leadership (1969–70). In C. B. Strozier (Ed.), *Self psychology and the humanities: Reflections on a new psychoanalytic approach* (pp. 51–75). W.W. Norton & Company.

Kohut, H. (1985b). The psychoanalyst and the historian. In C. B. Strozier (Ed.), *Self psychology and the humanities: Reflections on a new psychoanalytic approach* (pp. 215–223). W.W. Norton & Company.

Kulka, R. (2010). The contribution of self psychology to the spiritual dimension in psychoanalysis: Reflections on Heinz Kohut's self psychology and the humanities. *Ma'arag, the Israel Annual of Psychoanalysis*, *1*, 263–279.

Kulka, R. (2019). To study and to teach psychoanalysis. In T. Tamir-Oron (Ed.), *The theory and practice of the instruction of psychoanalysis in the psychoanalytic institute* (pp. 268–273). Israel Psychoanalytic Society.

Chapter 1

Captive in a Disaster

October 2023

Introduction

"Inflamed Nerve"[1]

Zion, in the beginning of my letter,
I'll ask about your well-being, how you feel,
All is well?
And how are your prisoners?
Your Palestinians?
Your Jews

Say, how are the children?
And how are your abductors, Zion?
Zion, won't you ask
for my well-being?

I don't feel
too well.

My right hand forgot its cunning, its nerve inflamed
Don't ask.

– Shva Salhoov

I am writing this chapter amid the horrific disaster.

One morning, a patient came into my office after we had both heard the news about the disaster that occurred during Israeli fighting in Gaza. Twenty-one Israeli soldiers were killed by the accidental discharge of explosives that they had put around the building they were sleeping in to protect themselves.

1 The English translation of this poem by Shva Salhoov, originally in Hebrew, has been sourced from Yeshurun and Lachman (2024).

DOI: 10.4324/9781003449386-1

When they were attacked by Hamas, the explosives ignited and caused the building to collapse on top of them. They were all killed.

The patient began the session by telling me about a thought she had at night: If she had lived at the time of the Holocaust, would she have hidden as a Christian, or would she have escaped? And if she had been a child in a concentration camp, would she have devoted herself to helping others and focused her energy on self-preservation, or would she have run to the wire fence knowing that doing so would have meant certain death?

The catastrophic events of October 7, 2023, and the war that erupted immediately after the attack caught us all by surprise, exposing Israel to a cruel reality worse than anything we could have imagined. Israeli society suffered a narcissistic blow unmatched since the establishment of the state. Hamas and terrorists from Gaza invaded the kibbutz settlements along Israel's border with Northern Gaza, overran supposedly secure Israeli outposts, and destroyed many residential communities, leaving a trail of devastation behind them, including hundreds of corpses. Simultaneously, other Hamas terrorists attacked a large outdoor music festival, called Nova, nearby at Re'im. Wherever the invaders went, they murdered, burned people alive, raped women, mutilated bodies, and beheaded many of their victims. They kidnapped 230 people – babies, young children, men, and women of all ages, including several elderly in their eighties.

In the days and weeks that followed, in border areas in the south and north of the country, hundreds of thousands of Israelis were displaced from their homes because of daily missile attacks. The Israeli soldiers, sons and daughters of many of us, were ordered to turn the territory of Gaza into a heap of ruins. According to estimates published by the United Nations as of the writing of this paper (August, 2024), approximately 40,000 Palestinians - Hamas fighters and non-combatant civilians, including a large number of children, were killed since the beginning of the war. Despite the devotion of the soldiers and their determination, there is clear evidence that this is a malignant experience for their bodies and souls. How do they return from this tormenting war? And what will be the fate of the Gazan people who are humiliated en masse, bereaved, injured, and uprooted? Do we sacrifice our future?

Two devastated people in a shared tragedy (Figure 1.1).

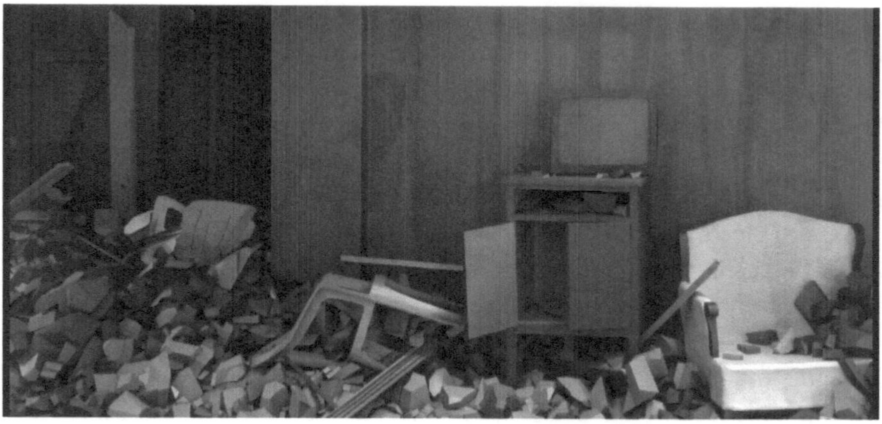

Figure 1.1 Thomas Demand's photograph titled "Ruin," captured in Gaza in 2014, was recently featured at the Israel Museum as a representation of destruction, embodying both the specific and the universal aspects of ruins within the Israeli context.

Source: Ruine/Ruin, 2017, C-Print/Diasec, 180 × 300 cm. © Thomas Demand, VG Bild-Kunst, Bonn

In Israel, the sense of "home" has been seriously undermined. Most of the country's citizens are experiencing a crisis of trust, no longer sure that the country's government and armed forces can provide basic security, the bedrock of everyday life. Questions about the future of both an internal and external "home" deeply disturb everyone's peace of mind. This disruption is particularly so when looked at from the perspective of the "fathers" (Israel's leaders) who have failed to provide safety for their "children." The fathers are viewed as having misled the public with unrealistic promises, blindness, and arrogance. Shortly after the attack, these same fathers announced to the public: "We will conquer them; we will crush them." In a dramatic voice, this message was repeated in the media every evening, even though the reality on the ground in Gaza could not validate this grandiose and tragic promise.

We may think of Laius, the father of Oedipus and king of Thebes, cursed by the gods. In his distress, and to prevent the fulfillment of the curse, he abandoned his innocent baby at the top of a bare mountain. He was not concerned with protecting himself and his future prosperity. He placed his personal good over the well-being of his son. This is how the stage was set for the subsequent tragic events. A father failed to assimilate his own past failures and violently projected his toxic mental contents onto the soul of the son, the other. The son and the citizens of Thebes were the victims of this tragic attitude.

The Israeli government failed not only to protect its citizens from the attack but also to provide support and care to victims after the incident. In the absence of a reliable "parental" presence in taking care of the war's injured and displaced, many Israeli citizens have become "parental children," selfobjects to one another, sorting out what the parents are unable to provide. While narcissistic parents are busy protecting their own interests, the parental children expend their best efforts to reduce, if only gradually, the consequences of the disaster. Among other things, what is especially evident is the remarkable mobilization of mental health professionals as volunteers to reach out to all those affected. This dedication to aiding others promoted a common human spirit among us.

In this chapter, I focus on those who are not direct victims; those who are exposed to the great magnitude of the disaster through relatives, their professional involvement, or who have been drawn voluntarily because they have special skills to attempt to identify who are the hostages and where they are being held by closely examining photo and video images of ghastly situations. In the literature, symptoms found among such people are termed "secondary trauma." However, one can readily see that the injury is not necessarily of secondary proportions. It is a trauma that impacts all Israelis. The world they believed in collapsed. A deeply held belief in basic security turned out to lack a foundation.

The events of October 7 and the months that followed ignited all our primordial anxieties. We met the evil gods face to face. Death stared at us from wherever we looked: the civilians and soldiers who were murdered on October 7, the soldiers who were killed in combat, the living and dead who were kidnapped, thousands who were severely injured, and the hundreds of thousands of Gazans who were displaced and humiliated en masse. This is a growing disaster that is difficult to contain in one's mind.

From the point of view of our professional concerns, this collective trauma is a comprehensive narcissistic injury whose expression can take different forms. Among some people, it can be expressed in the mobilization to help others, where mental resilience and resourcefulness are evident. Among others, there emerges a sense of fragmentation, a debilitating pain, a collapse into sadness and exhaustion, doubt in the essence of existence, mental freezing, and psychosomatic symptoms. We also observe displays of grandiosity and omnipotence arising out of a need for revenge, which is intended to restore the shattered cohesiveness of the self.

These contradictory self-states exist side by side and undermine the continuity of being. We are all captives of a disaster that assails the inner and external sense of homeliness, the body, and the mind.

In situations of environmental disaster and war, we analysts are required to deal with a complex issue: how to maintain a safe therapeutic framework, an appropriate sense of continuity and quiet conduct when the external reality rocks and invades the consulting room. In these circumstances, a unique transference relationship is formed between analyst and patient, a transference that is not permanent but varies from hour to hour and perhaps even within the same hour, depending on the immediate external and internal circumstances.

In a clinical diary that I wrote during these days of the war, I collected experiences from various encounters.

A Soldier's Father

"The Place Where We are Right"[2]

From the place where we are right
Flowers will never grow
In the spring.

The place where we are right
Is hard and trampled
Like a yard.

But doubts and loves
Dig up the world
Like a mole, a plow.

And a whisper will be heard in the place
Where the ruined
House once stood.

– Yehuda Amichai

A patient comes to the clinic after the October attack and can only talk about his son, who has been called up to the reserves and is about to enter Gaza with the army. The patient says that he is beside himself, cannot sleep, and

2 The text of the poem has been sourced from Gluskin (n.d.).

does not understand why his son, who is a reserve soldier in his early forties and the father of three children, should again be in the army and must fight in this war. He has, after all, said the father, already contributed enough to the country during his previous army service. At the same time, the father believes that there is no doubt that going to war is what needs to be done to ensure our safety and to heal the deep wound. "We have to attack them, show them," he says. While he is sure that the army usually knows what to do, he doesn't understand why they keep postponing the ground invasion of Gaza. "The command echelon," he says, "isn't exhibiting determination," adding that "excessive caution creates an absurd situation: waiting instead of acting." The father mentioned that he is also angered by the fact that I (the analyst) am "among those who appear to be hesitant, spineless, one of those who don't know what to do." He describes as unbearable what he calls my "helplessness."

I pointed out to him the intolerable anxiety that he experiences at the thought of a ground invasion alongside the rage he felt due to the delay of that invasion. I made a point of showing him that he had highly conflictual feelings about what should happen. I also made prominent in our conversation his disappointment at the stance he attributed to me. The feeling that we were not on the same page was, for him, inexcusable. He repeats and explains that he sees my attitude as a failure, an inability to understand him. And if I am helpless, how can I help him? He feels that I have "abandoned" him. This becomes the focus of our discussion.

The conversation soon turns to first memories, countless childhood images that remind him of his parents' lack of interest and failure to support him in any way. He felt that he was practically invisible within his family. He thinks that these negative experiences evoked in him an exaggerated need to be resilient, immune to harm, and tough. His parents did not supply the parenting that would nurture an appropriate sense of grandiosity; they did not imbue in him a healthy narcissistic experience of joy and hope. Low self-esteem and vulnerability led him to abhor displays of weakness. This evolved into an isolated arrogance and the admiration of omnipotent people while he denied the deep sadness buried within. He realized that his parents had failed him.

I found myself stunned by his anger and saddened by his distress. I felt that he was negating the possibility that my subjectivity could be different from his and erasing my concern, which, in fact, was focused on his concern for his son. Kohut (1984) and Anna Ornstein (1998) refer to such states of anger in the analysis when the patient's narcissism erases the analyst's attitudes. They caution that this kind of assault on the analyst can provoke in the analyst a rejection of the patient, mental fuzziness, and even aggression. The analyst's capacity to listen can be impaired, and her reactions might become false and superficial as a way of concealing her disapproval of the patient.

We were facing the possibility of being trapped in a major empathic impasse. We were on the verge of repeating his parents' refusal to cultivate resilience and encourage his healthy grandiosity.

I understood that the expectation that he would accept my subjectivity is fitting for someone who has a cohesive self and is capable of accepting otherness. However, he is in an archaic state and needs a selfobject that will validate his subjectivity, not mine. He needs recognition of the way he sees the situation. I thought about Kohut's (1972) suggestion to relate to grandiosity, even when defensive, in a welcoming manner and the need to supply the patient with a sense that he has efficacy. We know that patients do not easily give up unmet needs from their past; they continue to demand their fulfillment.

I searched within myself for an appropriate empathic response to his sense of outrage. In the next meeting, I formulated the following sentence: "They have brought upon us a disaster that cannot repeat itself." The intervention was a statement that drew on an ultimate reality; it was suited to his subjective need for mirroring and, at the same time, was also congruent with my thinking.

Formulating an intervention that transcends duality and still depicts the situation accurately is a challenging task. We need an intervention that enables the patient to emerge from his narcissistic vulnerability and alleviate the vertical split that he is caught in to regain a lucid and expanded mind. We assume that his rageful attitude was derived from the fragmentation of the self, a split mind: On the one hand, he was captured in grandiose, archaic fantasies and revengeful rage. On the other hand, he suffered from an acute existential anxiety in facing the danger to his son's life. This danger was obviously intensified, given the reality of the war and the low self-esteem rooted in his past. Moreover, he was frustrated and upset with my inability to undo the split situation and offer relief.

As analysts, we engage in the practice of reflection that constitutes a transitional area for becoming, which goes beyond any particular subjective stance. Winnicott (1971), in his introduction to *Playing and Reality,* wrote:

"In writing this book around the subject of transitional phenomena, I find myself continuing to be reluctant to give examples. . . . the thing that I am referring to is universal and has infinite variety" (p. xxii).

It is interesting that with the passing of the weeks and the onset of the land invasion of Gaza, the patient was able to relate more to his and everyone else's vulnerability, as well as the need to accept uncertainty. I felt that my creating a link with his perspective, in the way it happened, was recognized by him as fostering his area of faith and reinforced the transferential connection to me, the analyst.

An Uncanny Event

"The Silence is Dead"

The Golem lashes out in the streets
trampling beneath him the dreams
of people fleeing
to unprotected spaces.

Go to sleep, my son, sleep hush
The dog is dead so he won't bark
The dog is dead everything silent
The silence is dead.

The vampires are black, decapitating
joy from the people.
Hearing the screams outside
of the depleted souls.

Go to sleep, my son, sleep hush
Your brother is dead, he won't scream
Your brother is dead, everything is quiet,
The silence is dead.

Minotaurs in the streets
a bounty of corpse-piercing pitchforks.
Blood gushed like a river,
No river here,
only blood gushing.

Go to sleep my son, sleep hush
Mother is dead don't scream

Mother died here quiet,
The silence is dead.

There are no monsters, here people
doing the same things
without signs and without wonders
tearing flesh into shreds.

Go to sleep my son, sleep hush
My dead child will no longer scream
the child is dead everything is quiet
The silence is dead.
– D. Dori (written after October 7, 2003).
Translated by Linda Zisquit

In my encounters with hi-tech volunteers working at the civilian operations center dedicated to locating missing persons and with filmmakers who volunteered to document the war, I came to see that their work exposed them to terrifying scenes: burned babies, severed limbs, decapitated corpses, images of pregnant women whose bodies had been mutilated, and worst of all, eyes reflecting terror, "images from hell," as one of the volunteers explained. These images were etched in the minds of those who had seen them. They could hardly be deleted and frequently evoked insomnia, somatic problems, and nightmares. I heard people reporting that they had dreamed, for instance, about "a child who disappears," "people invading my home," and "attempts to escape but on a three-wheel bike." Each of the dreams reflected pre-traumatic experiences that emerged in the present context, even if the person was no longer consciously preoccupied with them.

Others had a compulsive need to cling to the terrifying images and view them repeatedly. A young woman who survived the attack on the music festival watches the videos of the festival time and again and cannot stop thinking about why she saved a certain anonymous person in her car and not also somebody else. A volunteer who was involved in identifying missing persons could not stop himself from comparing photographs of the missing taken before the disaster and photographs of the same persons taken after the disaster, for example, "a girl who was wearing a blue dress in a photograph in the family's album taken before the disaster, compared with a photo of a girl in a blue dress after the disaster." Was it the same girl? he asked. The volunteer says that he is concerned about becoming immune to these images. On the other hand, he feels somewhat apathetic when seeing the images. However, when he sees videos containing Arab music from Gaza, his entire body is overwhelmed by a feeling of terror. "These are the images that stick in the mind. . . . I have a volcano in my head," he explained. The volunteer says that what upsets him is the fact that watching the videos, in a strange way, calms him.

> If you see [the images,] there is no need to imagine them. . . . There is nothing new under the sun; think about the pogroms in Kishinev. . . . Think about the Vikings. . . . Beheading has been a known practice since time immemorial.

I understand that he is thinking about his children and wondering what kind of world they will be living in as adults. He doesn't mention his parents, who survived the Holocaust. What he is doing now is researching historical acts of massacre.

I can sense the dream and its shattering.

The irresistible desire to repeatedly view these horrific images clearly affected the public through the local mass media, such as the nightly news programs on television. "A photograph or a video can have a greater impact on the course of a war than a fighter squadron," Gideon Lev wrote in *Haaretz* on December 6, 2023. The most startling images appeared in the first videos released by Hamas, showing the kidnapping of an 83-year-old woman, who perhaps was by then suffering from cognitive incapacity, waving to persons around her, or the video of Hamas dumping a semi-naked girl on a jeep while watched by a group of surrounding men. The videos cultivated the feeling that nowhere was safe, certainly not one's home.

Weeks later, news videos presented the return of small groups of the kidnapped from Hamas captivity. These videos stimulated an internal dialogue among viewers and eventually the wider public between the normative reality and the black pole of human experiences; the uncanny threat became real.

This image of 9-year-old Ohad Munder being returned from captivity (Figure 1.2) is just one example of a video that could have been taken from a horror series occurring on the fine line between life and death. The video images of a Hamas terrorist seemingly compassionately embracing his little captive are difficult to look away from because the mind struggles to digest what the eye sees in disbelief. Video images of this type were shown repeatedly and compelled the public to take part in a nightly encounter with

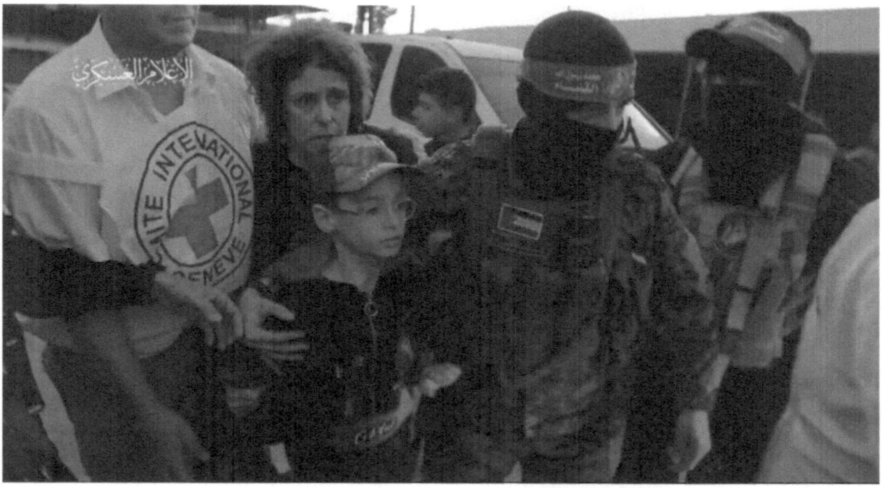

Figure 1.2 Ohad Munder's release from captivity, November 26, 2023.
Source: Creative Commons

the elegant but devious angel of death who was dressed meticulously. They depicted an encounter with a seemingly "humane" adult, who offered a bottle of water to the grandmother, while the mother, whose terrified eyes are riveting, grasps her young son. We, the public, increasingly felt obligated to participate in the sickening game that unfolded in front of us in the uncanny theater. It was a monstrous experience.

The thought that there exists, in reality, an underworld, and the king of Hades, the underworld, rules this world vigorously, as well as the images of Israeli soldiers walking in endless tunnels in this underworld with trained dogs in their search for the kidnapped hostages, also seems to be unreal. But knowing that the video is real creates the uncanny.

The concept of the "uncanny" appeared initially in a paper by Ernst Jentsch (1906), "On the Psychology of the Uncanny." Jentsch defined the uncanny as intellectual uncertainty or that which was undecipherable. In his 1919 paper "The Uncanny," Freud (1955) extended the understanding of the uncanny by emphasizing an emotional dimension in this experience. Analyzing Jentsch's work, Freud explained that it is possible to create an uncanny experience if one thinks of a wax doll, and a feeling arises at a certain moment that the doll may actually be real or that it could suddenly become an animate being. Freud was preoccupied with what was disturbing about these images. He characterized the uncanny as strange, threatening, mysterious, and incomprehensible. The word "uncanny" in German ("unheimlich") means "not homely," frightening because of the unfamiliarity. He wrote about the fascinating connection between the word "Heimlich" and the word *Geheimnis*, which means secret and is derived from the same root as *unheimlich*. Freud explained that when a secret (*Geheimnis*) exists within the home space, it transforms that space into an unhomely sphere.

One is reminded of fairy tales and computer games in which scary monsters and superpowers reign. We are usually sure that they are derived from the world of fantasy and therefore can be "domesticized." However, if these figures suddenly appear in reality, they will embody what Freud described as "uncanny." A sense of fear will be felt when what was perceived as a childish fantasy suddenly turns out to be more of a reality than we thought.

Drawing on his special insights, Freud explained what is found in the intensity of the uncanny experience: scary, repressed childhood memories are rooted in the depths of the unconscious. When a person encounters a threatening event in reality, the unconscious dread is triggered and becomes conscious. This is how childish fantasies of castration, the dangerous omnipotence of superheroes, aliens, and other threatening images turn into extraordinary experiences of horror and often create a process of compulsive repetition.

Using Winnicottian language, one could say that anxiety resulting from the mother's absence is tolerable if it does not go beyond X+Y minutes (Winnicott, 1971, pp. 95–103). It can be said that within this absence, the experience remains "homely." However, when the mother's absence lasts X+Y+Z minutes, Winnicott suggests that it may lead to madness. If we consider maternal presence as the fundamental essence of experiencing the "home," her overly prolonged absence turns the homely experience into an experience that is essentially unhomely and even uncanny. It can then constitute a basis for the fragmentation of the self: "Madness here means a break-up of whatever may exist at the time of *a personal continuity of existence*" (Winnicott, 1971, p. 97, italics in the original).

I wish to add here that another phenomenon that is relevant to the appearance of the masked Hamas terrorists is that of the "double." Freud (1955) notes that repeated appearances of the same object or being, in the same physical disposition, with the same gestures, but in different situations, produce an uncanny feeling. What could have been accidental becomes threatening, often creating an experience from which there is no escape. Freud pointed out that Otto Rank studied this phenomenon and linked uncanniness to silhouettes, to ghosts, and to anxieties about death. The idea of the double first appeared as a means of denying death. However, in ancient Egypt, when it was used to duplicate the images of the dead to signify the infinite afterlife, the meaning of the double changed from a promise of eternal life to the uncanny harbinger of death.

A bereaved mother

> A Monk asked: "The permanent – what is it?"
> Jōshū said, "That which is not permanent."
> The monk asked: "Why is the permanent impermanent?"
> Jōshū said, "Life! Life!"
>
> – Zhaozhou Congshen (1978, p. 43)

In one of my sessions during the war, a bereaved mother described in detail what happened the day there was "a knock on the front door."[3] Her children asked her many questions: Was it the daughter's hands that were wounded? Was it her legs? Did she die immediately or later? Did anyone come to her aid? These were questions she, in fact, also constantly asked herself. In my conversation with her, the mother focused on describing an event at one of the meals during the Shiva:[4]

> Suddenly, I noticed a brown butterfly that flew back and forth, back and forth, until it settled down on a chair. At the last meal, I again saw a butterfly, this time a white butterfly. I felt that she [her daughter] was with me.

In subsequent meetings, this bereaved mother talked about dreams she had about her daughter. In one dream, *she, the mother, is tasting some white cheese, and her daughter sticks out her tongue and wants the cheese, too.* She explained to me that sometimes they used to eat from the same plate.

3 The proverbial phrase "knock on the front door" is used to describe the moment when parents get the message that their son or daughter had been killed in a war.

4 The Jewish Shiva is a week-long period of mourning observed by bereaved families, during which they receive visitors in their home to offer condolences and support, reflecting on the life and legacy of the deceased.

Suddenly, a ginger cat appears in the dream and jumps onto her shoulder. She recounted further,

> I opened Google to see what the appearance of a cat in a dream signifies. Cats have mystical powers. . .; they symbolize feminine energy, a connection to the deep realms of intuition. They symbolize vitality, essentiality, the joy of life. . . . Here, the cat seized my daughter's place and grabbed the cheese. A cat is an animal that symbolizes fertility; they give birth to kittens often and in large numbers. . . . I jokingly told my husband, "I'm only 44 years old; we can have another child.

The mother commented, "It's not clear whether the cat is my daughter. Or did the cat take my daughter's life? Or is it the other child that we can still have?"

I remained in awe of the bereaved mother's ability to create in her mind an expanded space in which she could promote her reverie following her daughter's death. She was able to imagine her daughter's presence and also tried to come to terms with her absence. I appreciated her ability to understand the infinite potential of being. I noticed that in her dreams, whether daydreaming or night sleeping, animals appeared three times: a brown butterfly, a white butterfly, and a ginger cat. I thought that the brown butterfly was still a living butterfly and therefore signifies life. The white butterfly signifies death, and the ginger cat signifies excitement, energy. It may hint to the next incarnation of the daughter, the return of the potential to live, even if in a different way.

The colors indicated the changeability of self-states. The same can be said about the butterfly as an image because it also depicts transformability: first, an egg, then a caterpillar, a pupa, and finally, a butterfly. And, of course, we think of the myth that cats have nine lives.

Classical psychoanalysis treats dreams as an expression of repressed conflicts and distinguishes between overt and latent content. Dreams can also be comprehended as representations of the self-state. In this case, it is a visualization of a self that experiences a severe narcissistic injury and searches for transcendental avenues to cure the imbalance that is experienced. From this perspective, the mother can feel relief if she can constitute selfobjects, perhaps selfobjects that are virtual, for establishing a symbolic connectedness that would undo the existential disaster. The mother holds her child in an imaginary way that reduces the duality between life and death. This transformative work is her spiritual healing.

In his paper "On Courage," written in the early 1970s but published posthumously in 1985, Kohut mentions Sophie Scholl, who was a member of the German resistance movement during the Nazi regime and sentenced to death in 1943. On the last night before her execution, she dreamed that she was carrying a child in her arms, dressed in a long white garment, to be baptized. Suddenly, there was a crevasse gaping in front of her. She managed to deposit the child on the far side and then fell into the abyss. She explained that "the child is the leading idea; it will live on and make its way to fulfillment despite obstacles" (Kohut, 1985, p. 21). It is said that she faced her execution calmly and without a trace of fear. Her behavior testified to the total absorption of her idealized values. The dream embodied the courage of her nuclear self.

The bereaved mother, too, holds her daughter's representation within an evolving mind. Within the real dimension, the daughter is dead. However, from the perspective of an ultimate reality, the daughter is linked with her infinitely. One can, of course, suggest that the dream derives from a defensive need, but it is impossible not to see the transformative dimension, the touch upon the mystical in human existence. We notice the area of faith that lies beyond our conscious ability to perceive it by our senses. This expanded mind is, and will be in the future, prone to repeated fluctuations between moments of attachment to the concrete memories of being together with her child and moments of transformative reflection, in which her child has another existence within her.

How Can the Self Rescue Itself From the Clutches of Disaster?

The mind has mysterious ways of preserving terrible experiences and sometimes even getting trapped in them. One way is to create a vertical split that separates different experiences. In this way, one can focus on what is thinkable and divert one's gaze from other aspects of the situation, which are pain-producing. Rage is one instance of a one-sided perspective, a means of seemingly restoring the fragmented self. The rage provides a sense of control, resilience, and cohesiveness for a moment and erases the mental pain for a while.

These fragmenting processes are based on the exclusion of contents and not their integration. *Ex*clusion, not *in*clusion, is a process that limits the freedom of the mind. The self builds defense mechanisms for protection through denial, disavowal, and dissociation. Despite all this, inevitably, the shadows of horror will return in different ways. On the other hand, the mind can adopt transformative patterns that generate a perspective that transcends the immediate reality.

In our analytic work, it is of particular importance to validate the individual's particular traumatic experience. At the same time, and alongside the recognition of the particular subjective experience, it is possible to establish an understanding of the complexity of the trauma as an event that is not only one-dimensional. In the example of the father, it was evident that attachment to a particular identification and rage leaves the patient with an experience of loneliness and non-belonging. This is how the crack in the transference evolved. Inviting the patient to recognize the universal perspective and pointing out that which goes beyond the isolated personal mind offers him additional legitimacy and enables the establishment of awareness of a broader absolute reality. We saw that intervention of this type promotes the expansion of consciousness to a more complex perspective on the situation.

Another possibility is practicing the idea of transience. In my work, I often refer to the principle of transience, as Freud (1957b) first described it in his fascinating 1916 article "On Transience." He described a walk in the park with the young poet Rilke and the psychoanalyst Lou Salomé. Rilke complained that the falling leaves on a tree detract from the beauty of the garden. Freud explained that after shedding, spring would come, and the leaves would return. A year later, in 1917, he expanded his thinking on transience in his paper "Mourning and Melancholia" (Freud, 1957a). There, he already distinguished between healthy temporary mourning and melancholy, which leaves the person clinging to the shadow of the lost object. In any case, the idea of transience presents a significant change to classical psychoanalysis: instead of analyzing the past as a way to understand the present, the present is seen as holding the potential for the future. The present is a womb that will give birth to the future. It is about a possible evolution with a face to the future.

Another option I presented is the cultivation of the use of reverie. Imagination has the virtue of sending an anchor to other mental selfobjects that exist in a sphere that is beyond the immediate present, beyond what is known, beyond the frozen self-state, far from oneself, and from clinging to oneself. Within conditions of suffering, it is possible to discover realms of hope.

Marcel Proust (2020), in his book *In Search of Lost Time* (first published in 1914), mentioned the memory of his mother's Madeleine cookies as a recollection that restored the experience of the continuity of the self. In *Man's Search for Meaning* (first published in 1946), Victor Frankl (1959) described the memories of his mother's Friday meals as a way to find an anchor of meaning during his captivity in the concentration camps. These are connections to idealized selfobjects in virtual reality or in creative acts. Cultivating them can be formed within analytical treatment.

Winnicott opens his essay "The Location of Cultural Experience" (originally published in 1967) with a quote from Tagore: "On the seashore of endless worlds, children play" (Winnicott, 1971, p. 95). The mind expands when it places itself within an infinite potential space. The mind is no longer imprisoned within the inner life, not even in the happenings of the real world. Both are disaster areas. The mind, aligned within the potential space, can expand beyond the present and reach new realms from moment to moment and from day to day.

David Grossman testified that when his son, Uri, was killed in Lebanon, he was in the middle of writing *To the End of the Land*, first published in Hebrew in 2010. When he heard the "knock on the front door," he thought he would not be able to continue writing. But sometime after the son's death, the story began to pulsate in him, and he returned to writing. The need to preserve the image of the lost son only grew stronger. He longed to inject into his dead figure new life and vitality. He sought to bring his son back to life in the imagination. The act of creativity works against the gravity of mental pain. "If I was sent to this impunity," Grossman said in *Haaretz* in October 2023, "at least I'll give him my words; I'll let him resurrect in my imagination."

Creativity creates the world and makes it possible not to attach to a narrow-minded point of view. In an open state of mind, we have a higher chance of being able to listen, accept complex situations, and decipher their meaning without sinking into distortions. Here, the analyst's quiet attitude is important and her willingness to recognize the vulnerability that we all share, including her own vulnerability. The analyst's ability to remain in an equanimous state of mind must be established before trying to establish this position in the patient. It is the analyst who is responsible for cultivating the ability to see beyond immediate distress.

When the self is courageous enough to connect with the ultimate, it is in a transformative state that restores horizontal and vertical splits. The area of faith is constituted once again. This creates the possibility to transform archaic narcissistic vulnerability into a compassionate consciousness, which accepts vulnerability as part of man's destiny. Man finds selfobjects, real or virtual, which regenerate his vitality and creativity.

The world no longer closes.

Grossman wrote:

> Hope can be seen as an anchor, thrown out of a suffocated and desperate existence toward a better and freer future. Toward a reality that does not yet exist, most of which is made up of wishful thinking. . . . The anchor is thrown and clings to the ground of the future, and then the person, and sometimes an entire society, begin to pull themselves toward it. It's an optimistic act: the ability to cast the imaginary anchor beyond the tangible and arbitrary circumstances indicates that in the soul of the person who dares to hope, there is still one place that is free. A place that no one has been able to suppress, nor to pollute.
>
> (*Haaretz*, October 30, 2023)

References

Frankl, V. (1959). *Man's search for meaning (Revised and updated)*. Washington Square.

Freud, S. (1955). The uncanny. In J. Strachley & A. Freud (Eds.), *The standard edition of the complete psychological works of Sigmund Freud: Vol. 17 (1917–1919): An infantile neurosis and other works* (pp. 141–156). Hogarth Press.

Freud, S. (1957a). Mourning and melancholia. In J. Stachley & A. Freud (Eds.), *The standard edition of the complete psychological works of Sigmund Freud: Vol. 14 (1914–1916): On the history of the psycho-analytic movement, papers on metapsychology and other works* (pp. 237–258). Hogarth Press.

Freud, S. (1957b). On transience. In J. Stachley & A. Freud (Eds.), *The standard edition of the complete psychological works of Sigmund Freud: Vol. 14 (1914–1916): On the history of the psycho-analytic movement, papers on metapsychology and other works* (pp. 303–307). Hogarth Press.

Gluskin, S. (n.d.). *Days of awe* [Blog]. The place where we are right by Yehuda Amichai. Retrieved March 24, 2024, from https://daysofawe.net/shebotzodkim.htm

Grossman, D. (2010). *Ishah boraḥat mibeśorah [To the end of the land]*. HaKibbutz HaMeuchad Publishing House.

Jentsch, E. (1906). On the psychology of the uncanny. *Psychiatrich-Neurologische Wochenschrift*, *8*(23), 203–205.

Kohut, H. (1972). Thoughts on narcissism and narcissistic rage. *The Psychoanalytic Study of the Child, 27*, 360–400. https://doi.org/10.1080/00797308.1972.11822721

Kohut, H. (1984). *How does analysis cure?* (A. Goldberg & P. Stepansky, Eds.). University of Chicago Press.

Kohut, H. (1985). On courage. In C. B. Strozier (Ed.), *Self psychology and the humanities: Reflections on a new psychoanalytic approach* (pp. 5–50). W.W. Norton & Company.

Ornstein, A. (1998). The fate of narcissistic rage in psychotherapy. *Psychoanalytic Inquiry, 18*(1), 55–70. https://doi.org/10.1080/07351699809534170

Proust, M. (2020). *In search of lost time* (C. K. Scott-Moncrieff & S. Hudson, Trans.). RMB.

Winnicott, D. W. (1971). *Playing and reality*. Basic Books.

Yeshurun, H., & Lachman, L. (Eds.). (2024, January 28). Ten seven. *Curated: Thinking with Literature*. Retrieved March 24, 2024, from https://arcade.stanford.edu/content/seven-ten-two-look-straight-our-eyes

Zhaozhou Congshen. (1978). *Radical Zen: The sayings of Jōshū* (Y. Hoffmann, Trans.). Autumn Press.

Chapter 2

Seeing Beyond Blindness

On the Link Between Kohut's and Bion's Transcendental Psychology

Introduction

Not-knowing is not just an individual occurrence. We are all too familiar with group blindness in situations of social violence, blindness to the plight of its victims, and blindness to the pleas of opposing groups. A blind attitude helps us to escape social responsibility and avoid pain. It enables the individual to remain innocent and unaffected. We may consider it as our task, as mental health providers, to support individuals and groups in finding ways to transform blindness both in analysis and beyond. During the evacuation of the Gaza Strip by the Israelis, a compelling phenomenon erupted. We witnessed hundreds of people who truly believed that the evacuation would not occur in spite of overwhelming evidence to the contrary. On August 19, 2005, the day of the evacuation of Neve Dkalim, an Israeli civilian settlement in the Gaza Strip, I found the following report on the front page of *Haaretz*, which described a group of women in the synagogue of Neve Dkalim:

> It is doubtful that any of the young women had entered the hall during the day without noticing that Neve Dkalim was no longer there; even when Rabi Shlomo Aviner gave his blessing . . ., they wouldn't believe it was all over. They refused to accept the evacuation and had turned their heads away from the glass door and the windows, through which one could see the enormous battalions that had started to dismantle the men's stronghold in the Sephardic Synagogue at the other side of the courtyard, and that will soon be easily evacuating them too. And when they started to sing, "God, hear my plea," the song came to a halt, this time with cries of dread. The troops had broken into the hall.
>
> (*Haaretz*, August 19, 2005)

DOI: 10.4324/9781003449386-2

We may wonder what motivation could be so powerful that these women preferred not to see the reality as it unfolded in front of their eyes. What could have explained their willingness to be totally unprepared when the moment of evacuation arrived? Was it simple denial, a wish not to know? Or should we regard this state of mind as an attempt at transcendence, an attempt to create an alternative reality by a total reliance on the power of belief in God? While we may not ever be able to formulate a simple answer, it is clear that emotional blindness leads to human tragedy and suffering.

The Phenomenon of Not-Knowing

Three universal myths relate to the problem of knowledge. In the myth of Eden, the challenge consists of not eating the apple from the Tree of Knowledge. Transgressing this prohibition brings about shame and expulsion from paradise. In the Babel myth, curiosity and excessive thirst for knowledge are represented by constructing a tower that would reach heaven. God, unwilling to let the people reach these spheres, decides to confuse their language and destroy their communication. Finally, in the myth of Oedipus, his relentless quest to uncover the truth by any means becomes the dominant force that results in tragic consequences.[1] The common element of the three myths is a search for knowledge in the face of its being forbidden and a lack of intuitive wisdom to judge what should be known and what is beyond knowledge.

An essential part of our humanness seems to involve our continuous grappling with what can be known. Our shared, profound dilemma is that knowledge may be obstructed in some circumstances, or it may emerge in others; it takes various forms and transformations. Meaningful knowledge is attainable only within a positive link (+), a context in which two people or two parts of a mind – or mind and body – are related positively to each other. However, where intolerable anxiety, fear, envy, or shame is evoked within such a context, a negative link of knowledge will evolve. In this case,

1 The paradox of knowing and not-knowing has preoccupied mankind from the beginning of civilization. To "see" means "to understand"; it reflects the link between seeing and comprehending. In the myth of Oedipus, gouging out the eyes means relinquishing "external sight" for the sake of constituting internal profound comprehension. The prophet Tiresias, in this tragedy, validates this perspective: the blind prophet is not inspired by false external events but sees the ultimate truth.

meaning is denuded of vitality so that discovery and development become impossible. There will be no function for discriminating between true and false. The result of such an intersection will be, in some cases, the proliferation of lies as a barrier to truth (Grinberg et al., 1993). Bion believed that truth is a permanent source of pain and that the human being's capacity to tolerate truth about himself or herself is fragile. The tendency toward evasive action is great, and the mind is always prepared to create lies to oppose the pain.

Another configuration that relates to not-knowing (or emotional blindness) is the phenomenon Bion (1984a) called "reversal of perspective." This originates in the well-known experiment in perceptual psychology that consists of the observation of a print that can represent either a vase or two profiles. He uses this experiment as a model of all situations of insight in which the person can switch from one point of view to another in relation to what is happening. The capacity to tolerate paradox provides a basis for mental creativity and development. In distinction, reversal of perspective is a complex phenomenon in which the individual tends to remain in one perspective only, from which he or she "sees" the reality. This is not a manifest attitude; on the contrary, it hides behind an apparent agreement and understanding.

In practice, we encounter situations where it appears that patient and analyst understand each other and are in agreement, but, in fact, they do not make any transformative contact. Interpretations remain repetitious and empty. We may consider this situation a defensive organization formed to operate against awareness.

Kohut (1971) also depicted such a one-sided attitude when he proposed the radical idea of the vertical split. He posited that narcissistic needs that remain with no sufficient response foster a fragmentation of the psyche, a *vertical split*. In contrast to the *horizontal split*, which refers to repression, one finds the coexistence, side by side, of incompatible psychological attitudes ranging from slight incongruence to a situation that verges on fragmentation. We may see the manifestations of unmodified rudimental grandiosity side by side with manifestations of a self that is bound to realistic goals. One attitude is blind to the other. Kohut (1972, p. 385) elaborated the description of such a state of mind further in his extensive discussion of the narcissistically injured person's rage: the narcissistically injured, on the other hand, cannot rest until he has blotted out a vaguely experienced offender who dared to oppose him, to disagree with him, or to outshine him. For Kohut, narcissistic rage is an indication of suppressed, unmodified narcissistic needs, which become intensified as their expression is blocked. Such states often coexist with emotional blindness.

It is both Bion's and Kohut's understanding that such cases of fragmentation indicate not only that the contained is unable to use the container productively but also that the container fails to respond to the emotional needs of the contained/subject. Bion relates to this inability to learn from experience as a – K link.

In Kohut's terms, we could say that the selfobject is unable to lend itself creatively to the self's needs. In many cases, this is an intensification of frustration in the connectedness between self and other, a lack of oxygen, in Kohut's words. This empathic failure disturbs the narcissistic balance, constituting defensive accommodations in the relation between the self and the other. We can assume that the subject, who experiences an environment that fails to know him or her, eventually gives up the wish to be known. Such an unmetallized experience might be extruded from the mind and evacuated into the body, into intersubjective experiences, or into the trans-subjective sphere (Puget, 1995), the realm of action and social violence.

While we relate to the patient's resistance to uncover the truth during the analytic process with some understanding as an expected variable, we also continually must consider the less recognized resistance put up by the analyst to the evolution of insight and intuitive knowledge. The analyst has his or her own anxiety, which warns of dangers and the high prices of coming face to face with the patient's catastrophes. In the interaction between patient and analyst, the patient's projections may induce unbearable feelings in the analyst. The analyst, being unaware of what is happening, feels bewilderment and unease and may be unable to tolerate it. At this point, the analyst may violently reject the material or displace his or her reaction in some way so as to disguise it. The analyst may evacuate discomfort by resorting to action in various forms.

Therefore, it is important to talk about the vicissitudes in the patient's and analyst's different states of mind: *Both* patient and analyst have a blinded mind and an illuminated mind. The blinded mind comes to the forefront in an uncontained context, provoking defensive acting and the preference not to see. In contrast, the illuminated/creative mind is guided by a free flow of intuition, contains the pain, and carries out the analytic work. Thus, it is vital that we consider both the intrasubjective interaction between opposing factions within each person's mind and an intersubjective relationship between two people. The context is what determines which part is brought out.

Clinical Vignette

A short clinical vignette will illustrate the process of transforming blindness in the therapeutic encounter. The material was presented to me during supervision by a therapist who works in a center for the treatment of victims of terror and war. The patient was a young woman doing public service (in place of army service) in Tel Aviv. She called the hotline of the center after a terrorist attack in Tel Aviv and complained that she suffered from excessive anxiety, fear of being attacked, and difficulty in sleeping. She was referred to therapy.

The patient comes from a religious settler's family in the West Bank. Her background was instantly conveyed by her code of dress: long sleeves, long dress with long pants underneath. The therapist noticed her pretty eyes with their sad expression. She disclosed immediately that she was doing a period of state-sponsored public service against her mother's will and was not sure whether this was the right decision for her. However, she needed to distance herself from the family. She believed that God was probably putting her on trial for separating herself from her family's wishes or was punishing her. She also made it clear that she did not know what psychotherapy was about but that, given her current discomfort, she was willing to try it out.

Consider the following interaction within its social context: severe political stress between the religious right-wing settlers of the occupied territories and the "lefties" who are opponents of the occupation. This vignette took place after a year in which the patient had become incredibly committed to the process of therapy.

There was a long silence, which was unusual for her. The therapist felt that there was a barrier between her and the patient, that she wanted to say something that was hard for her. The therapist mirrored this feeling to her. The patient confirmed her therapist's notion and mentioned that she was very angry with her instructor at work, who criticized her. She described what happened: She had to give children a lesson about Rabin's assassination[2] and read his autobiography to them. When she came to the Oslo agreement (a partial peace agreement between Israel and the Palestinians),

2 The Israeli Prime Minister Yitzhak Rabin was assassinated in Tel Aviv on November 4, 1995, at the end of a rally in support of peace and anti-violence. In his remarks at the rally, Rabin declared that he always believed that most of the people want peace and are ready to take a risk for it. The assassin was Yigal Amir, an Israeli law student and radical right-wing nationalist who opposed the Oslo peace initiative.

she inserted the following sentence: "In this agreement, Rabin gave the Palestinians weapons to kill *my* neighbor." The therapist tried to understand whether she was talking about a specific event. The patient explained that this was not a concrete event. It was the intention to kill "all" her neighbors: the Jewish people in the settlement.

The session took place on Rabin Memorial Day itself (November 4). The therapist felt revolted, flooded by rage and pain, and was aware of the growing distance between her and the patient. When she tried to encourage the patient to elaborate more on what she thought, the patient began to present extreme right-wing ideology, which was even more upsetting to the therapist. The therapist reported that she was close to breaking out of the therapeutic setting and involving herself in a harsh political discussion or interrupting the session at once, yet she controlled herself and mumbled a few sentences about who is a victim and who is an aggressor. When the session was finally over, the therapist felt confused between the outer reality and psychic reality; she felt immense anger and revulsion toward the patient as well as guilt and disappointment with herself for failing to contain the situation better.

The therapist said she waited eagerly for the supervision hour. It was the first time she had brought this case to supervision. As soon as she started to report the hour, I articulated my feelings to her: "There is a feeling of catastrophe here; your patient is in great turbulence, and you could not find compassion for her; it must have touched a painful string in you."

Following this intervention, the therapist spontaneously unfolded her personal subjective experiences of pain. She recalled her father, who had died two months before. Her father was a Holocaust survivor who wanted to build a better life for himself and the generations to come. As a victim of racism in various concentration camps, every manifestation of violence was unbearable for him. He adored Rabin and his efforts to bring peace. The therapist grew up absorbing these values.

The therapist then shared with me that her birthday is actually on the day of the Balfour Declaration, a statement by the British government in 1917 regarding their intention to establish a home for the Jews in Palestine. She let that show as the carrier of this declaration and that she was committed to it. There was a pause in our dialogue, and she suddenly said:

> The patient and I actually share a common element. We were both born in an unsafe place. Both of us are actually exposed to a similar sense

> of catastrophe; I am concerned about what will happen to the state for which my parents fought bitterly, and she is threatened about the future of the territories where she grew up all her life.

Now we could comprehend that the patient's pain and her own pain were not so different. It was a moment of encounter with the foundations of each person's deepest fears and mental pain and the constitution of the patient's subjectivity.

Rather than having been attuned to the patient being a victim of circumstances that happened prior to her birth and later on, the therapist now realized that she had seen her patient as an aggressor who was out to destroy her own fundamental values. She had taken the patient's distortion of Rabin's story at face value, from one single perspective with no elaboration of its subjective meaning. As the supervision hour proceeded, the therapist recalled how the patient was born after the death of her grandfather and how her depressed mother never held her in her arms. She was an unheld baby born on shaky territory. When she read the text to the children, she was struggling to maintain both her internal home base and her actual house, which was about to be destroyed. Moreover, the therapist's premature intervention and lack of attunement prevented the patient from safely elaborating on her suffering and pushed her toward a defensive position. The long-lasting rift between the patient and her inattentive mother was reenacted in the session, this time vis-à-vis the therapist.

The realization that each of them had her own spiral of traumatic personal history enabled the therapist to understand her empathic failure. She recognized how her own dread obstructed her ability to feel compassion for the patient. She understood that external reality and psychic reality were conflated in her mind for a while. The supervision created space to see the underlying narcissistic injuries both of the therapist and of the patient and to transform this knowledge into a transcendental vision of suffering. The supervision hour ended with an expectation that unfolding the impasse would provide both patient and therapist with an opportunity for further growth. This transformation was only superficially connected to the overt content of the hour. Rather, it was related to the therapist's ability to touch on the underlying spheres of the mind and its subjectivity.

Two weeks later, the patient expressed a wish to attend therapy sessions twice a week. She now reported a dream which she defined as a "Holocaust dream" in which "faceless people are marching with suitcases in their hands." In her associations, she referred to the future evacuation of her settlement; she was offering a pictorial image of her internal catastrophe, the sense of her home collapsing and the shaky ground. Finally, she articulated clearly, "One day, my home will be taken away forever, and what will I be able to retrieve?" Then she added, "The sad thing is that people think about this in terms of ideology. They do not understand the suffering involved." The therapist was astonished: Was the patient now dreaming the history of her own father? In her mind, a faceless patient, labeled "the settler," had become a real person: Ester.

This vignette demonstrates a situation in which a containing function and sufficient empathic echoing transform impersonal phenomena and dogmatic thinking into truly subjective experiences. The supervisor's role as witness and container was transformative in the sense that it allowed the therapist the possibility of holding on, thinking about, and "digesting" problematic and painful materials. A link of knowledge (K+) was established. Let us bear in mind that Bion portrayed the container-contained link by symbols that imply the existence of a sexually productive pair. In such a context, new meaning can be conceived. In the present example, a "now moment" occurred in the sense that the therapist suddenly realized something that was previously blocked out of her mind. If we think once more about the experiment in perceptual psychology, the therapist was suddenly able to see an alternative perspective. In Kohut's terminology, we can assume that a vertical split was restored.

More so, the transformation that occurred for the therapist enabled the quick renovation in Ester's mind, too: She was no longer in a defensive position that drew her into blind ideology; she could let herself emerge and unfold. We may think about Kohut's (1984) notion of the selfobject's function in balancing the empathic matrix.

But there is more to it. The vignette illustrates a moment of encounter where blindness is transformed into a broad vision beyond the realm of intersubjectivity. When the therapist suddenly realized that she and her patient had something in common, that they were both born in an unsafe place, a transformation of a different order occurred. I, as a supervisor, realized that some radical change occurred in the therapist's mind. Dissolving the most complex boundaries between them, as therapist and patient, as representing right- and left-wing schools of thought enabled the therapist to transcend to a different state of mind that is beyond knowledge. The therapist gave up the exclusive commitment to her own subjectivity and her own single-perspective version of history. She was no longer an exclusive self in itself.

At once, she felt compassion toward *all* those who were forced out of their places and whose environment was unsafe, regardless of their affiliation.

I believe that, in our example, my comment to the therapist provided her with a "background of safety" that enabled the spontaneous change in her state of mind. She did not need to defend herself, nor did she feel guilt or shame for what seemed like a lack of containment on her part. She immediately relinquished her narrow perspective of the patient. In place of that, she retrieved compassion toward herself and could now unfold her own subjective experience and make the unexpected leap to the transcendental mode. The patient responded to the shift in her therapist's mind and changed the setting to twice a week. Then she presented the "Holocaust dream" with a supra-intersubjective significance in regard to all the uprooted. Ester made her own leap into the transcendental realm.

A narcissistic capsule, in which the therapist was captive, transformed into a broad vision of human fate. Once this freedom of sight was attained, a state of serenity that consists of reconciliation was achieved, and the richness of the therapeutic encounter was now allowed to unfold freely. What we are talking about is transcendental transformation that can occur when compassion is allowed to emerge.

In Buddhist texts, the concept of compassion is often connected to situations of animosity, not to situations of love. Compassion is not necessarily a function of positive emotions; it is the ability to be in another person's place, often in his or her suffering or pain or in his or her different modus. In our example, this happened twice: first, when the therapist said, "I realize that we have so much in common," and following that, when Ester brought her "Holocaust dream," a visual image that encapsulated her fate, the therapist's personal history, and the suffering of *all* the uprooted. Furthermore, she later elaborated and said: "The sad thing is that people think about that as ideology. They do not understand the suffering." She recognized now the defensive and blind nature of her own ideology.

One question remains open: Can such transcendental transformation extend beyond the rooms of the therapy? To answer this question, I would like to refer to an additional incident between the therapist and Ester that occurred a year and a half later, during the civilian and military withdrawal from Gaza in August 2005. During this period, extremely high tension was felt all over the country. Right-wing people at this point wore orange shirts or used orange flags to signify that their suffering was reminiscent of the Jews forced to wear the yellow star when they were forced out of their homes during the period of the Nazis. Left-wing people used blue and white flags and condemned the right-wing comparison between the Israeli disengagement from Gaza and the Holocaust as utterly absurd.

At one session during his period, Ester entered the room and left her backpack outside. The therapist asked why she did not want to bring it into the room. Ester said that it was too heavy. The therapist offered to help her, and they both carried the bag into the room. Ester mentioned that she had come from Meimon (a violent demonstration of settlers against the disengagement). The therapist wondered whether she had an orange shirt. Ester responded: "My shirt is in the bag. I left the bag outside; orange is not needed in this room."

"Orange" is a symbol of narrow vision and is now mindfully kept ex-territorially out of the room. Ester chose to leave the dogmatic mode of being outside of the room when meeting with her therapist. Did she totally relinquish the "Orange Mode" as an act of transcendence, or was she trying to disavow the conflict when being in the presence of her therapist, inducing a split between various circumstances? We cannot be certain, yet I believe that the creation of an ex-territorial space for her therapy is a manifestation of trans-contextuality (similar to what Winnicott meant by transitional phenomenon), not a function of a split-off animosity. Thus, the therapeutic achievement is that she realized that she could be different in different contexts; in certain contexts, she chooses to eschew "orange." She has become mindful enough not to wave the "orange" flag around in an undifferentiated manner. This is an act of transcendence by itself.

Do transcendental experiences contribute to the relinquishing of the "orange mode" in situations beyond the therapeutic situation? Is the therapeutic encounter adding to the emergence of compassion and serenity beyond? I can offer only one response. We need to hold on to such faith.

Expansion of the Mind: On the Transcendental Psychology of Bion and Kohut

This example illustrates how the role of a container or a selfobject[3] is transformative in the sense that it allows the subject a possibility to

3 The container provides the subject with a place to repose its feelings so as to transform them or use them as a communication. The selfobject, on the other hand, lends itself to the self, immerses itself in the self, and enables the self to emerge from its virtual form to cohesion.

hold on, think about, and "digest" problematized and painful materials in the presence of another. It illustrates moments of encounter where the narrow mind is transformed into an expanded mind that has broad vision.

At this point, we should mention the radical move of both Bion and Kohut beyond the notions of their original schools in the realm of object relations toward transcendental psychology. In 1965, Bion coined the concept of transformation in O to represent a process of becoming, of intuiting the unknown, and moving toward an underlying truth (Bion, 1984b). Becoming O is possible only if a state of "at-one-ment" is allowed to take place; the analyst can achieve the mental frame in which he or she can be receptive to O only if he or she has the capacity to be in "at-one-ment" with it. It could be equivalent to empathy but seems more complex (Lopez-Corvo, 2003). It is a form of relating where open intuition is tuned toward a communion with truth. Bion drew his concepts from the world of mystics, who were known to perceive an inner illumination, which they described as a union with God (Symington & Symington, 1996). For Bion, the godly revelation of the mystic was similar to the revelation experienced by the psychoanalyst while mindfully listening to the patient and bearing him or her in mind. At a certain moment, the moment of "at-one-ment," something is understood and liberated from emotional blindness: first within the analyst, then within the patient.

Kohut illustrated the various forms and transformations of narcissism. In its sublimated fashion, one can think about "cosmic narcissism" (Kohut, 1966, p. 266), a perspective that bears an important correspondence to Bion's thinking about O. In certain circumstances, if the cohesive self is secure enough to relinquish its personal narcissistic goals, it can dissolve into a new psychological configuration, far removed from any previous personality structure; it can transcend to cosmic narcissism, a state of "supra-individual participation in the world" and expanded sense of self merged within the world. It has to do with a dissolved state of selfhood, beyond cohesion and beyond structure: a state of interbeing and nonseparation from the broader surrounding. It refers to those unique and cherished moments when individual narcissism is transformed into an amalgam of higher experiences of belonging. Kohut (1966) points out that this is not a new state of being hurt but rather a return to the "original psychological universe, i.e. to the primordial experience with the mother" (p. 266), when the self was bound with her, namely was beyond itself.

Bion's concept of "at-one-ment" and Kohut's notion of cosmic narcissism may be regarded as moments of ultimate interconnectedness, which necessitate that both container and selfobject need to empty themselves of their memory, desire, and previous understanding (Bion, 1988), as well as their own prominent modes of operation and their narcissistic positions. It is not that they need to be literally empty but that they need to be willing to relinquish holding on to their usual tendencies and attitudes. Letting go of their individual and mutual motives allows for a free-floating mind to work in the hour and beyond. Bion (1988) phrased such an attitude quite radically: "The psychoanalyst should aim at achieving a state of mind so that at every session he feels he has not seen the patient before. If he feels he has, he is treating the wrong patient" (p. 19). Such high levels of experience are beyond the utilization of projective identification and intersubjectivity. The relevance of projections as a mode of communication is on the wane. Transcendence is a different order of communication.

Such an attitude enables compassion: daring to see painful parts of reality and not pushing them away, accepting parts of others and of ourselves that are not the ones we necessarily like. What is implied is not being fixated on a dogmatic experience, not being caught up in our own version of reality; instead, maintaining an open space and freedom to feel and experience a whole range of emotional states. This notion puts an emphasis on contextuality, on being realized by all phenomena.

Conclusion

Let us return to our starting point: Neve Dkalim. One question still remains open: Are the transcendental transformations in analysis, which we perceive as creative extensions of the mind, equivalent to holding on to transcendental positions, such as illustrated by the tragic story of Neve Dkalim? While I will probably fail to answer this question comprehensively, we have to bear in mind one substantial difference. Ester was able to dissolve her protective narcissistic shield since she was securely held and positively mirrored by her analyst. Not needing to hold on to her old means of self-protection allowed for a fundamentally different experience, an immanent transcendence and mindfulness that stemmed from the inner freedom that she gained.

In the story of Neve Dkalim, the opposite was true. Here, a dangerous situation evoked unbearable anxiety and fears of nonexistence, with no adequate contextual containing or selfobject support. In a way, it resonates with Bion's description of ignorance and arrogance. It is a state of mind that tries at transcendence to a different reality, to create an alternative reality by a total reliance on the power of self-conviction.

To put it in other words, in the story of Neve Dkalim, anxiety was dealt with by organizing around the sense of collective continuity and singularity, by creating an illusion that "we" exist, will continue to exist, and have a privileged position of existence. Constructing and continually reconstructing this collective "we" gravitates against the painful realization of truth. It is a dynamically charged ignorance that seems like a narrowing of the perspective rather than an extension of the mind. Most significantly, it is an attempt to be redeemed by an external miracle, not a function of inner freedom or resilience. Such transcendence has to be distinguished from transcendental experiences. In transcendental experience, enlightenment derives from within.

As analysts, we have to consider the unique significance of immanent transcendental thinking. As people who think about cure, we ask ourselves, what is that ultimately brings about psychic growth and the optimal unfolding of the self? I believe that states of transcendence, when we rise above concrete and discrete analytic materials, are the moments in the analytic setting when we gain authentically new perspectives and that these moments are the highest manifestations of an expanded mind. In such moments, containing and empathy evolve into compassion. We are then able to free ourselves from preconceptions, seeing beyond the immediate while bringing about change that has a fundamental distinctive quality.

What exactly allows for a universal awareness at a certain moment is unknown. This kind of awareness cannot be easily explained or justified by particular processes or special concepts. Its quality can be described only as a sense of connectedness with a broader sequence of events that is there at a particular moment.

When do such moments occur? Only experience can provide an answer to this question.

References

Bion, W. R. (1984a). *Elements of psychoanalysis*. Karnac Books.

Bion, W. R. (1984b). *Transformations*. Karnac Books.

Bion, W. R. (1988). Notes on memory and desire. In E. B. Spillius (Ed.), *Melanie Klein today: Developments in theory and practice: Vol. 2: Mainly practice* (pp. 17–21). Routledge.

Grinberg, L., Sor, D., & Tabak de Bianchedi, E. (1993). *New introduction to the work of Bion* (Rev. ed). J. Aronson.

Kohut, H. (1966). Forms and transformations of narcissism. *Journal of the American Psychoanalytic Association, 14*(2), 243–272. https://doi.org/10.1177/000306516601400201

Kohut, H. (1971). *The analysis of the self: A systematic approach to the psychoanalytic treatment of narcissistic personality disorders*. International Universities Press.

Kohut, H. (1972). Thoughts on narcissism and narcissistic rage. *The Psychoanalytic Study of the Child, 27*, 360–400. https://doi.org/10.1080/00797308.1972.11822721

Kohut, H. (1984). *How does analysis cure?* (A. Goldberg & P. Stepansky, Eds.). University of Chicago Press.

Lopez-Corvo, R. E. (2003). *The dictionary of the work of W.R. Bion*. Routledge. https://doi.org/10.4324/9780429481482

Puget, J. (1995). Psychic reality or various realities. *The International Journal of Psycho-Analysis, 76*(Pt 1), 29–34.

Symington, J., & Symington, N. (1996). *The clinical thinking of Wilfred Bion*. Routledge.

Chapter 3

Paradoxes of Belonging

Introduction

This chapter presents a picture of an Israeli who is trying to solve the riddle of her fragmented identity and heal a rupture in the self: "Who am I?" "Where do I really belong?" "How do I cultivate a broad perspective on immediate contradictory self-states?" These are profound questions for many Israelis. Motivated by the wish to retrieve a secure experience of belonging and connect to a nontraumatic transcended sense of self, the taking of a spiritual journey opens up a path toward compassion and a profound understanding of the complexities of belonging and identity.

Two vignettes illustrate such transformation. The first vignette is a personal account that portrays the ruptured self of persons who were expelled from Germany and settled in Palestine. While relieved that they had found a new haven and shelter for their plagued selves, they experienced an unrestorable breach in their identities and in their sense of belonging. The vignette portrays the first generation's complex connectedness to Germany and the second generation's search for the lost link. The second vignette is a discussion of a segment from the film *Waltz with Bashir*, a cultural icon exploring current Israeli identity. This vignette focuses on the split self-experience of an Israeli soldier who is called to serve in the army and to fight in Lebanon while he, the perpetrator, deeply identifies with the victims who, in his mind, remind him of his refugee parents.

Vignette I: A Personal Account

My knowledge about my father was incomplete. I knew that he was a young professional in Germany when his office in Königsberg (now Kaliningrad,

DOI: 10.4324/9781003449386-3

Russia)[1] was confiscated one night by the Nazis, and he was put in jail for "shaming the race." It was never clear to me what "shaming the race" meant until many years later, when he was 82 and my mother had died. One Friday night, he came over as usual for dinner, excited and emotional. He said he needed to consult with us. He pulled out a tiny passport picture of a young woman. He told us that she was his fiancée back in Germany and that he had been arrested because of his relationship with her and forced to leave Germany. She had wanted to join him in Palestine, yet his father was against it; "Germans cannot come to Palestine," he said. So he lost her in oblivion until one day he received a letter from her. This was in the 1960s when he was working in Israel as a lawyer, making claims in the names of Holocaust survivors for restitution from Germany. She was the secretary in one of the law offices in Germany with whom he corresponded. In her letter, she wondered if he was the person she knew back in Königsberg. Until that time, she had been certain that he had perished. This renewed contact was soon lost again until many years later when my mother passed away, and she communicated with my father again. The question then was whether he wished to meet her once again. She was in her seventies; he was in his eighties.

My father asked what I thought. Should he meet her, or should he preserve the memory of her as she was when he knew her in Germany? He hesitated for several months; finally, he wrote to her that it was better to leave things as they were. The letter came back undelivered. She had died in the meantime.

When he was 93, and the borders to the Russian exclave of Kaliningrad were opened to tourists, my father asked me to visit his hometown with him in Königsberg. When we arrived there, we wanted first to go to his former home, but we could not find it. The Russians had destroyed most of the prewar housing. Ironically, however, the Russians preserved the train station and the very platform from which my father had been deported. Generally, however, there were few traces of the past. My father wanted to find the church in Königsberg where he secretly had met his lover. There

1 Königsberg, a historic city founded in the 13th century in Prussia, became Kaliningrad following World War II. After the 1945 Potsdam Agreement, the city was annexed by the Soviet Union and was renamed in 1946 after Mikhail Kalinin, a Soviet leader. Today, Kaliningrad is an exclave of Russia, situated between Poland and Lithuania on the Baltic Sea, retaining its strategic military and economic significance.

was no church. Finally, the taxi driver mentioned that there is a residual of a church, a single arch, at the edge of a parking lot. We went there. My father recognized the church setting; it was on the bank of the river he remembered very well. He had played there as a child.

My father said, "*Even the Nazis and the communists could not take my river away*." I should add the following: As a child of Jews who were forced out of Germany, I grew up in a German-speaking house, yet it was a "faux pas" to speak German in public at that time in Israel. I did not speak German for more than 30 years. In 2005, I was invited to participate in a conference in Dresden, Germany and to conduct a group discussion for three days in English. The participants were mostly Germans. After the first day, I started to speak a bit of German. On the third day, I conducted the group in nearly fluent German. One of the Germans in the group was an analyst. She was not only the same age as me and shared the same psychoanalytic orientation, but as it turned out, our grandmothers are buried in the same town in Germany, Essen. We realized something else; our mothers sang the same lullaby to us: "Guten Abend, Gute Nacht." In a fleeting moment, I felt that we have common ground, in spite of belonging to "opposite sides" of the very tragic historical event that was formative for each of us, in different ways.

It was impossible not to recognize that our personal histories are intertwined in a mysterious way. It was not just our age, womanhood, motherhood, and professional interests that connected us but an unspeakable intuition that we belong to the same catastrophe. I felt that we might well have been school comrades were it not for the catastrophe that caused my parents to flee Europe. These events intrigue me, and I am still not sure that I can comprehend their full meaning. I think about the unexpected finding that I, a native Israeli, and my German colleague belong to very different worlds. Yet there is an endless intercourse between my subjective becoming and hers. We talked, and often we still talk about our families and the "thing" that connected us so strangely. Comprehending the full meaning of this endless entanglement between our shared destinies requires an act of faith.[2]

2 Winnicott (1971), in his introduction to *Playing and Reality*, writes:

> This paradox, once accepted and tolerated, has value for every human individual who is not only alive and living in this world but who is also capable of being infinitely enriched by exploitation of the cultural link with the past and with the future. It is this extension of the basic theme that concerns me in this book.
>
> (p. xii)

Vignette II: An Israeli Soldier

Waltz with Bashir is an Israeli animated documentary film written and directed by Ari Folman. It depicts Folman in search of his lost memories from the 1982 Lebanon War (Halkin, 2009).[3] In 1982, Ari Folman was a 19-year-old infantry soldier in the Israel Defense Forces (IDF). The year is 2006, and in the film, he meets with a friend from his army service period, who tells him of a recurring nightmare connected to his experiences from the Lebanon War. Folman is surprised to find that he does not remember a thing from that period, not even the night of the Sabra and Shatila massacre. His only "memory" is a hallucinatory vision of himself and his soldier friends bathing at night by the seaside in Beirut, in what looks like a primordial-infinite sea, under the light of flares descending over the city. Folman embarks on a cinematic quest for the forgotten past. He cannot find words, images, or any appropriate language for describing his experiences in the war. He is

---

Kulka (2003), in his introductory essay to the Hebrew edition of *Playing and Reality*, elaborates this view:

> Man is defined both as an imminent and a transcendent entity. This is to say, man is a finite and an infinite creature, this is the essence that life consists of . . . at any point in time. Whereas traditional psychoanalysis defined men through their imminent qualities and regards development as the relinquishment of illusion and mature mourning, Winnicott presented to psychoanalysis a radical attitude that consists on the idea of continuous creation of life and the world.
>
> (p. 12)

3 In June 1982, following the collapse of a year-long truce between Israel and the Palestinian Liberation Organization (PLO), the Israeli army invaded a Lebanon torn by years of civil war. It did so after the PLO, which controlled much of the Lebanese south and had its headquarters in the western half of Beirut, had directed rocket and artillery fire at northern Israel. The PLO, for its part, was responding to an Israeli air strike on Beirut, carried out in retaliation for an attempted Palestinian assassination of the Israeli ambassador in London. The Israeli government had made no secret of its belief that a showdown with the PLO in Lebanon was inevitable; rumors had circulated widely of a military alliance with Lebanon's Christians, whose main militia, the Falange, was led by a pro-Israeli politician named Bashir Gemayel.

Folman's unit was in the Lebanese capital in mid-August, when the siege ended with the capitulation of the PLO's forces and their expulsion to Tunisia and was still there in mid-September, when Bashir Gemayel, the pro-Israeli newly elected president, was assassinated. In the aftermath of his death, revengeseeking Falangists, on an IDF-supported mission to flush out remaining PLO fighters from the Palestinian refugee camps of Sabra and Shatila, massacred close to a thousand of the camps' inhabitants. Soon afterwards, Israel was harshly criticized for its alleged role in the massacre, both from the outside and from inside; 400,000 people gathered in Tel Aviv to protest against this occurrence, refusing to let this tragedy pass unnoticed. As a consequence, Israel withdrew from the Beirut area, and the war was effectively over.

The movie depicts a soldier who finds himself in the midst of this terrible massacre.

searching for a curative context that will help him regain his lost memory and understand what had happened to him. He speaks to a psychologist he knows; looks up old army buddies who were with him in Lebanon, travels to Holland to find one of them; visits a specialist on post-traumatic stress disorder; and talks to an officer whose men were a short distance from the refugee camps when the massacre took place. Finally, he interviews Ron Ben-Yishai, the first Israeli reporter to enter the camps the morning after.

As he goes relentlessly from interview to interview, Folman finds his self-experience gradually restored. From this point on, *Waltz with Bashir* moves back and forth – indeed, "dances" – between Folman's reawakened memories and the accounts of his interviewees. The film ends with Folman's memory of the night of the massacre. He was one of the Israeli soldiers who were firing mortar flares from a rooftop to illuminate the camps for the Lebanese Falangists who massacred the residents of the camps of Sabra and Shatila. From up there, they could see the long lines of Palestinian women march slowly and mutely out of the refugee camps.

At that moment, he regains insight. He comprehends that there is a deep uncanny connection between these marching women and him; his parents marched like that as well in other times, in other camps. These women are not as foreign as he wished to believe. In this last scene, the animation alters into actual footage of the aftermath of the massacre, murdered Palestinians, shot by the Falangists, lying in bloody heaps. This, says the film, is the reality into which the audience is asked to awaken before leaving the theater. This is the private reality into which Folman has awakened as well. He now looks at the catastrophe from a new compassionate perspective: it is the victims' catastrophe, and he too is one of the victims; the "objective" division between victim and victimizer, Israelis and Palestinians, does not hold anymore. This lucid realization makes it possible for him to regain his lost sense of humanness and repossess his identity.

We can assume that the vision of bloody heaps of the dead represents the actual catastrophe as retrieved in his memory but also signifies unbearable guilt in which the hero is now helplessly captured. Thus, the awakening that takes place is twofold: it lifts the horizontal split, the repression of unthought known fault, opening up a possibility of reparation, and at the same time, it heals a vertical split – that between the innocent humane self and the disavowal of humaneness. As long as those splits are maintained, no mental pain can be experienced, and no reparation is possible. Now that it is possible to conceive of the complexity of these thoughts, the injured self can be transformed. The hero, and probably the audience too, assumes responsibility for the loss of humaneness and recognizes the subjectivity of the suffering stranger (Orange, 2011), as well as their own subjectivity.

The questions "Who am I?" "Where do I really belong?" and "How does one cultivate a broad perspective on contradictory self-states?" are profound ones for many Israelis. What has happened to the "Beautiful Israeli," the one who was characterized by an enormous passion for building a haven/heaven for the Jewish people, the one whose identity was consolidated and whose destiny was well defined? What is continuing to happen within the mind and heart of the contemporary Israeli who must, on the one hand, defend her place and, at the same time, be exposed to the constant risk of losing her virtue in this process? How can we incorporate the oscillations between being children of refugees who lost everything and being fighters who, at times, become entangled in ethical dilemmas that seem to disavow our own past as refugees? Do we sometimes yearn for our lost, unfractured sense of belonging and wish to regain it?

The Israeli is trying to decipher the manifestations of the past in the present and assimilate conflictual dimensions so as to heal profound vertical splits. The search for the past – whether it is our family's history, our parents' traumatic experiences, or our own – is an attempt to repair a weighty rupture of the sense of belonging. The wish to understand this rupture is not just an ordinary investigation of the past in the Freudian sense of uncovering that which is repressed. Nor is it a search for integrating good and bad internalized objects in the Kleinian sense. Rather, it is an exploration of lost potential and its retrieval, "*re*membering" that which is *dis*membered, still disavowed; that which could have been there, yet remains unconstituted, bringing it out to be part of an enriched, cohesive, healthy identity. It is a quest that requires and encompasses a compassionate search for a lost internal home of safety.

Theoretical Considerations

Kant (2007)[4] made the distinction between noumenon and phenomenon: The noumenon is one thing, one elemental entity, *the* substance; the phenomenon is multiple, a series of manifestations of such substance. The

4 Symington (2012), in his lecture "Psychoanalysis: The Noumenon Contrasted with the Phenomenon," describes the true nature of psychoanalysis and uses Kant's distinction between noumenon and phenomenon to distinguish between its manifestations and its substance.

noumenon consists of a profound awareness of an ultimate reality, much like Bion's (1984a) O, whereas the phenomenon is a particular aspect of such ultimate reality. The noumenon does not create any divisions and consists of a non-dual perspective, as opposed to the phenomenon that changes according to contextual conditions. Therefore, personal experiences are minute bits and pieces of broad past histories and futures that stretch for endless years. Through various phenomena, we try to come in contact with the hidden noumenon to broaden our mindfulness to that which is at the heart of our existence.

Kohut (1966) searches for the underlying nature of things, their "nuclear essence" or their virtual quality and the way things are prior to their pathological-destructive twist. He relates to that self-state, which is experienced with the mother primordially, the "original psychological universe" when the self was safely bound with her. The theoretical assumption is that the child's unruptured identification with the mother must be regarded as a precursor of a search for interconnectedness and wholeness later in life. People "remember" such primal experiences and yearn for them (Ghent, 1990). For Kohut, such connectedness is the normal and most meaningful state of being (Strozier, 2001). Kohut elaborated on this idea when he introduced the term "cosmic narcissism." He refers to infinite transformations of narcissism. He defines it as a state of participation in a "supra-individual" existence, an extension of the self beyond its particular boundaries, the ultimate transformation of narcissism. This perspective does not contradict personal narcissism in its various forms.

This perspective – albeit in different variations – can be found in current self psychology writings. For example, Orange (2008) writes: "We share a common humanity – with all its potential for good and evil – and are the other to each other, the You that meets the I in mutual dignity and reverence" (p. 120). Sucharov (1992, 2001, 2013) writes about wholeness and its healing qualities: "When we fully embrace complexity and wholeness, we encounter a glimpse of the infinite totality of which we are part" (Sucharov, 2013, p. 393). In the same paper, he summarizes the ground rules of complexity theory:

> Complexity systems theory tells us that by virtue of our continuous being in the world, we all stand, at any given moment, at the center of a complex totality of experience that is informed by multiple and interweaving contextual systems. While one can say that every moment is sacred for

> its unique and irreducible complexity, there are certain moments in one's life that bring into the foreground hitherto unexamined connection.
>
> (p. 381)

John Riker (2010) suggests that transformations of narcissism consist of a universal extension of ethical concern. He noted as much in a 2011 paper:

> The full ethical position demands that we extend our empathic concern to others with whom we are not in [a] reciprocal relationship, that we give respect to all human beings and maybe all sentient creatures. . . . The choice not to extend empathic, respectful care to all human beings . . . involves a fragmentation of ourselves.
>
> (p. 111)

Further on, he states: "When I retain the essence of myself . . . regardless of circumstances, then I actively assert my being in the world" (p. 113).

Writing about the transformative perspective, Kulka (2012) believes that we may renounce a particular form/manifestation for the sake of a transformative position. In fact, we oscillate between our self-experiences as individuals and our self awareness of being part of a vast humane entity. Even though we need to realize that this transformative perspective is not part of the mainstream of psychoanalytic thinking, such distinction between the particular individual manifestations and the search for an underlying common existence is at the heart of major psychoanalytic theories, such as Winnicott's (1971) concept of potential space and Bion's (1984a) concept of O. It is a zone of potentiality that recognizes the profoundly curative qualities of the ultimate reality, the primordial nature of things, that which existed prior to conflict and rupture. Finally, Frie and Coburn (2011) regard the contextualized nature of human experience and the sense of belonging as essential elements that heal the isolated self. There is a yearning and a need to feel and experience a sense of belonging, "being human among humans," as Kohut (1984, p. 200) indicated.

Healing the Fragmented Self of the Israeli

Israelis are experiencing circumstances that are related to isolation, alienation, conflictedness, and self-states that consist of paradoxes of belonging. Israelis may be entangled in war situations that they did not wish for; they may feel disconnected from traditional and Zionist values; they may feel that basic ethical standards that are fundamentals of the Jewish state are not enforced enough; they may wish to disentangle themselves from the constant oscillation between being a "victim" and being a "victimizer"; being a "proud" Israeli versus being a "shameful" Israeli. They may feel a profound rupture between phenomena that occur in their daily lives and the foundations of their heritage.[5] Obviously, they may also identify with the need to protect their country to maintain its freedom and security. This Israeli self, being wounded by a continuous chain of traumatic events, oscillates restlessly between different fragments of its fractured identity.

Let us assume that this wounded self is not an isolate, nor is it a fixed entity. If so, we need to consider the idea that the same self may in different circumstances present with different manifestations. These different manifestations, however, are part of one elemental self. This is because the sense of isolation and the need to shield the self arise at any moment in a certain context and may disappear in a different context. In certain circumstances, the self may seem to be split, fragmented or disintegrated, blocked, frozen, deformed, and rigid; it tends to hold vast areas of experience at a distance. Yet, in other contexts, this very same self may be creative, spontaneous, vivid, and open to an infinite realm of experiences.

We may assume that vast parts of the creative self are not lost but held up, derailed, or disavowed. The primordial, radiant self is there and can emerge at any time if the conditions are right. It is reasonable to assume that there is an everlasting yearning to regain and realize this pre-traumatic vast potential.

As analysts, we lend ourselves to our patients and strive to offer them a lucid view that perceives the ultimate reality and recognizes profound entanglement. To do so, we have to cultivate our own ability to transcend our tendency to gravitate toward particular individual phenomena instead of experiencing the ultimate dimension. Here, the concepts of equanimity, empathy, and compassion are important (Mann, 2013a, 2020), including the cultivation of our own compassion as analysts to see and accept the vast complexity of self-experiences.[6]

5 In the summer of 2011, the thousand protesters in Israel coined the concept "The new Israelis." They called for a return to the fundamental ethical values of the state of Israel, its innocent raison d'etre.

6 In the Kiddush, a prayer that is said on Friday before Shabat, one thanks God for having "chosen us (the Jewish people) out of all nations." Lately, this sentence has been changed, in some circles, and people thank God for having chosen us (the Jewish people) as all nations.

In each and every hour, we may focus on chronic disappointments and losses, those that occurred yesterday and which may or may not reoccur tomorrow. At the same time we may open our hearts to that which is unknown, new, not yet born in our mind. When we engage in unstructured meditative listening, we may see the potential that has not surfaced yet. It may emerge as a natural sphere of the self. We try to restore the wounded self in a way that will restimulate its missing vitality and regain its lost potential.

By touching this dimension, we help our patients widen their constrained sense of belonging and identity. Touching this seed of spirituality brings the self back to its natural habitat.

Return to the Vignettes

If I may go back to my own memories for a moment, I think that my German colleague and I managed to do something that my parent's generation was unable to do. My parents' generation had difficulty in imagining any link between the world that deported them and their present world. My father had obeyed his father when he left his fiancée behind to travel to Palestine, and later on, as an old man, the idea of integrating his past into the present by establishing contact with his former lover promised too much of a storm to try to act on it. Yet he spent his life working on restitution for Holocaust victims, and when he came to the end of his life, the trip to his hometown restimulated an existing link and partial reconciliation: "Even the Nazis and the communists could not take my river away." At that moment, I understood that he could reestablish a link with his childhood territory to retrieve his innocent sense of belonging to this childhood nature. However, he could not reconcile with the people who belong to this primordial world. I was taken aback by the liberating quality of his statement; here, there was some realization of the endless chain of possibilities that go beyond individuality and time to something broader and more enduring than the fragility of the impermanent particular self.

My colleague and I were able to remove the dark side of our common history from the heart of attention without disavowal of it. As friends, colleagues, and analysts, we were able to accept different facets of the same crystal, respecting and tolerating the paradox of "separateness and union" (Winnicott, 1971, p. 99). I believe that *for both of us*, this unique connectedness is expressed in a search for a lost link.

Ari Folman, too, embarks on a personal voyage to bridge gaps in his sense of belonging and identity. Here, the use of animation plays a major artistic role. Forman depicts the common wish not to know and the courageous struggle involved in the attempt to uncover his painful experience of belonging. Folman totally lost his memory; what remained was almost a hallucination that mystified and idealized the real events.

Yet we can also look at Forman's situation from a different angle. The animated pictures reflect fairy-like approximations of reality in the best way possible for the injured self. That which really occurred cannot be presented, spoken, or even thought about when the self is not sustained by an empathic selfobject context. We create a fictional story about the real story when no one is there to maintain an emphatic matrix to immerse with; when there is no one there to share these experiences of the self. We eliminate details or fabricate details with regard to the phenomena not merely out of a defensive motive but more so out of our vulnerability and incapacity to face the truth when totally alone.

The relentless struggle to uncover the elemental identity persists due to a profound need to purify the self of its distortions, from its projections, vertical splits, and from perversion. The hero is looking for an area of faith (Mann, 2010), a healing context to cure a deep deficiency. This curative endeavor is possible only in the presence of a compassionate selfobject, who agrees to share and re-experience these memories with the self. In *Waltz with Bashir*, the hero engages his friends and the audience to re-experience the events with him and re-experience the painful complexity (Brothers, 2008). In this sense, retrieving memories is giving back to the self its cohesiveness, its virtual pre-traumatic qualities, and its innocence (Felman & Laub, 1994[7]; Ornstein, 1994[8]; Eldridge, 1997).[9]

7 Felman and Laub (1994) link trauma as experience outside the range of comprehension; it is blindly repeated until someone bears witness to the story that "cannot be witnessed" (pp. 68–69). Memories happen through testimony.

8 Anna Ornstein (1994), referring to Kohut, writes:

> Kohut helps us to appreciate the fact that it is not possible to understand the inner world of an individual in the therapeutic situation without placing that individual in the particular historic – cultural context in which he or she grew up.
>
> (p. 132)

She continues and suggests that structuring the narrative of memories is a process that structures the self, contributes to the reestablishment of self-cohesion, and heals the vertical split between experiences as they are lived and as they are remembered. Finally, she argues that retrieved memories will be accompanied with deep sorrow and grief, indicating that the increase in self-cohesion makes it possible to accommodate that which previously threatened the self with fragmentation.

9 Amy Eldridge (1997) writes: "The therapist and the patient must co construct a meaningful narrative in which these memories are able to undergo structural transformation and become elements of the patient's self-experience" (p. 83).

Indeed, in *Waltz with Bashir*, all objective occurrences remain marginal for a long time; the emphasis is on subjective reality. Folman, much like any ordinary patient, searches for interpretations of his dream-like experiences and at the same, he creates insights and new understanding for others. Thus, he is not only a "patient" who strives to restore his own fragmented self but also the "analyst" who asks questions and promotes understanding and the unfolding of new meaning. He transcends any particular role in favor of a universal quest for a cure. In fact, he even engages the audience both as "patient" and as "therapist" at the same time. In this artistic endeavor, the audience becomes part of this extended expedition to uncover their hidden selves, retrieve humaneness, and purify the intoxicated self. The animated scenes that finally transform into double-edged documentary materials portray the move to a lucid comprehension of human destiny. The hero is no longer alone; a healing context of forgiveness is found.

I wish to conclude with a quote from David Grossman's *New York Times* article "Writing in the Dark" from 2007:

> I write. I relieve myself of one of the dubious and distinctive capacities created by the state of war in which I live – the capacity to be an enemy and an enemy only. I do my best not to shield myself from the just claims and sufferings of my enemy. Nor from the tragedy and entanglement of his own *life*. Nor from his errors or crimes or from the knowledge of what I myself am doing to him. Nor, finally, from the surprising similarities I find between him and me.
>
> All of a sudden, I am not condemned to this absolute, fallacious, and suffocating dichotomy – this inhumane choice to "be victim or aggressor," without having any third, more humane alternative. When I write, I can be a human being whose parts have natural and vital passages between them, a human who is able to feel close to his enemies' sufferings and to acknowledge his just claims without relinquishing a grain of his own identity. . . .
>
> We write. The world is not closing in on us. How fortunate we are.

References

Bion, W. R. (1984a). *Transformations*. Karnac Books.

Brothers, D. (2008). *Toward a psychology of uncertainty: Trauma-centered psychoanalysis*. Analytic Press.

Eldridge, A. (1997). Walking into the eye of the storm: Encountering "repressed memories" in the therapeutic context. *Progressive Self Psychology*, *13*, 69–84.

Felman, R., & Laub, D. (1994). *Testimony: Crises of witnessing in literature, psychoanalysis and history*. Routledge.

Frie, R., & Coburn, W. J. (Eds.). (2011). *Persons in context: The challenge of individuality in theory and practice*. Routledge.

Ghent, E. (1990). Masochism, submission, surrender: Masochism as a perversion of surrender. *Contemporary Psychoanalysis*, *26*(1), 108–136. https://doi.org/10.1080/00107530.1990.10746643

Grossman, D. (2007, May 13). Writing in the dark. *The New York Times*. www.nytimes.com/2007/05/13/magazine/13Israel-t.html

Halkin, H. (2009, March 1). The "Waltz with Bashir" two-step. *Commentary Magazine*. www.commentary.org/articles/hillel-halkin/the-waltz-with-bashir-two-step/

Kant, I. (2007). Ground of the division of all objects into phenomena and noumena. In M. Weigelt (Ed. & Trans.), *Critique of pure reason* (pp. 251–263). Penguin Books.

Kohut, H. (1966). Forms and transformations of narcissism. *Journal of the American Psychoanalytic Association*, *14*(2), 243–272. https://doi.org/10.1177/000306516601400201

Kohut, H. (1984). *How does analysis cure?* (A. Goldberg & P. Stepansky, Eds.). University of Chicago Press.

Kulka, R. (2003). Radical continuity in psychoanalysis (in Hebrew). In D. W. Winnicott (Ed.), *Playing and reality* (Hebrew ed., pp. 9–30). Am Oved Publishers.

Kulka, R. (2012). Between emergence and dissolving: Contemporary reflections on greatness and ideals in Kohut's legacy. *International Journal of Psychoanalytic Self Psychology*, *7*(2), 264–285. https://doi.org/10.1080/15551024.2012.656357

Mann, G. (2010, October). *The domain of non-duality: An area of faith*. Presented at the 33rd IAPSP Annual International Conference on the Psychology of the Self, Antalya, Turkey.

Mann, G. (2013a). Being human among humans: Response to Maxwell S. Sucharov's "Thoughts on wholeness, connection, and healing: Moving toward complexity in the analytic space". *International Journal of Psychoanalytic Self Psychology*, *8*(4), 398–411. https://doi.org/10.1080/15551024.2013.825946

Mann, G. (2020). Emptiness, equanimity and the selfobject function. *Psychoanalytic Inquiry*, *40*(5), 300–310. https://doi.org/10.1080/07351690.2020.1766321

Mann, G. (2015). Paradoxes of belonging. *International Journal of Psychoanalytic Self Psychology*, *10*(3), 275–286. https://doi.org/10.1080/15551024.2015.1043844

Orange, D. (2008). Psychoanalysis in a phenomenological spirit. *International Journal of Psychoanalytic Self Psychology*, *4*, 119–121. https://doi.org/10.1080/15551020802527845

Orange, D. (2011). *The suffering stranger*. Routledge.

Ornstein, A. (1994). Trauma, memory, and psychic continuity. *Progressive Self Psychology*, *10*, 131–146.

Riker, J. H. (2010). *Why it is good to be good: Ethics, Kohut's self psychology, and modern society*. Rowman & Littlefield.

Strozier, C. B. (2001). *Heinz Kohut: The making of a psychoanalyst*. Farrar, Straus and Giroux.

Sucharov, M. S. (1992). Quantum physics and self psychology: Toward a new epistemology. In A. I. Goldberg (Ed.), *Progress in self psychology* (pp. 199–211). Routledge.

Sucharov, M. S. (2001, October). *The infinite, the sacred and contextualism*. Paper presented at the 24th Annual International Conference on the Psychology of the Self, San Francisco.

Sucharov, M. S. (2013). Thoughts on wholeness, connection, and healing: Moving toward complexity in the analytic space. *International Journal of Psychoanalytic Self Psychology*, *8*(4), 379–397. https://doi.org/10.1080/15551024.2013.825944

Symington, N. (2012). The essence of psycho-analysis as opposed to what is secondary. *Psychoanalytic Dialogues*, *22*(4), 395–409. https://doi.org/10.1080/10481885.2012.700872

Winnicott, D. W. (1971). *Playing and reality*. Basic Books.

Chapter 4

Perpetrators and Victims

Can the Self Renounce Its Trauma?

Introduction

"Arrival"[1]

Gray fog
Covers the horizon
. . . fresh air! A relief
Chimneys?! . . . A factory?! . . .
"Don't delay! Don't
look for your belongings,
get into a line!"
"You Jew!" You are alive . . .
only work awaits you?!

Women to this side!
Give their children to their
grandparents, quickly
Groups form . . .
Where shall you stand?
What will be "good"?
Your husband goes to the left
There . . . Selection!
The Mission?
Ask the man in the uniform! He may understand
Don't be shy!

. . . It's impossible . . .
shall you hide? He shall look

1 Ornstein (2004, p. 67).

DOI: 10.4324/9781003449386-4

at the masses . . . only at the heads.
On your head
quickly a red scarf. Young,
not forced smile . . . Life
wants to live.
Into five!
. . . No noise . . . no commotion
Only the fog and the silence
outside. Inside the
thoughts can't find their places.
What's the smell?
Does it burn someplace?
And then the
Knowledge and the Terror combine.

– Anna Ornstein (2004)

The aftermath of the Holocaust has left large sectors of the survivor community – the children of survivors and the children of persons who died in the Holocaust – mentally imprisoned. Many of these trauma victims are brutally deprived of the psychic freedom necessary to fully flourish as human beings. As Hannah Arendt has so vividly written, the concentration camps were the penultimate inversion of life, second only to death. A life-arresting trauma has quite clearly been passed on to the second and even third generations, many of whom live in Israel. Psychoanalysis and psychotherapy in Israel are centrally concerned with attempting to liberate the second and third generations from the inherited shackles of the Holocaust.

This chapter describes the analytic work of a group of Israeli–German analysts who have explored their personal histories and analytic cases with each other for 14 years. The group began with a strongly felt split between "perpetrators" and "victims" – "German" analysts and "Israeli" ones. We assumed that the members of each group carried suffering linked to the Holocaust, whether overtly or concealed. And then we learned in our many sessions together that second-generation Germans are in different ways imprisoned by their Nazi past, though of course not in the same way or with the same intensity that survivors and their offspring are imprisoned by the remains of the Holocaust. The group consisted of members of the Institute for Psychoanalysis in Heidelberg, Germany, and members of the

Contemporary Institute of Psychoanalysis in Tel Aviv, Israel. The meetings occurred annually, alternating between Tel Aviv and Heidelberg.

The purpose of our work was to investigate whether working together in a group setting could facilitate dissolving malignant internalized identifications and finding ways to free oneself from the grip of trauma. We hoped that opening ourselves to the descendants of persons on the other side of the trauma would help us find a common humanity despite our profound differences.

The analytic process, even though stressful at times and always challenging, led to a deepened understanding of how our fates are affected by the same historic event. We are all children of a deeply injured generation, and we all carry complex identities related to this past. We realized that we have a common language derived from psychoanalytic thinking and a unique opportunity to discuss events, experiences, and memories that could not be discussed at all, or not fully, with our families and friends. We knew that the events and their aftermath were expressed in our lives in subtle ways in spite of the dearth of talk. We also agreed that we differ fundamentally in the sense that nothing can be compared to the suffering caused by the Holocaust.

The group experience offered each of us an opportunity to broaden his or her perspective and facilitated transformations. Eventually, our dialogue transcended conventional splits; we could share experiences of vulnerability and pain. It was possible to relinquish preconceived attitudes about each other and accept an ethical code of responsibility to explore and understand as much as possible what happened, as well as accept that much is incomprehensible. Accepting that the fact of incomprehensibility carried with it a sense of enhanced freedom.

The group started with six German members and 12 Israeli members. Six Israelis left the group at different times for different reasons (health, inability to cope with being in Germany, other commitments, emigration from Israel, and conflict with the group). We dealt openly with each of these losses.

The meetings were self-regulated by the members and had a fixed setting: The first session of the whole group was always called "Why are we here?" Thereafter, for two and a half days, the members met in different combinations. In "Group Together," all of the members shared their personal experiences and explored tensions as they arose. These tensions derived at the beginning from a lack of mutual trust between the Israelis and the Germans. Later, as trust grew, there were tensions not specifically related to the identities of the participants: tensions among "founding members" of each institute and younger analysts and tensions between the founders of the common group and other members of the common group.

In "Group Separate," Germans and Israelis met separately with members of their own groups. This was occasionally necessary to contain the tensions that emerged in the common group. Sometimes, it seemed that the differences between the groups were so profound that there was a way to bridge the gap. At other times, there developed internal tensions within each group, and these were also analyzed in the separate meetings. The separate meetings were used to try to transform such personal injuries into a more general understanding of cultural and personal differences.

Each year, we also presented four clinical cases: two Israeli analytic cases of second-generation patients and two German analytic cases of patients who grew up in German homes immediately after the war. We learned that often the atmosphere in the postwar German families was still informed by fascist principles and Nazi upbringing, cruelty toward children, strict boundaries, and fear of talking openly. We tried to depict these unique characteristics in these analyses. The last session was always "What do we do next year?"

As we approached the last meeting of the group, we decided to reflect on our subjective experiences in writing. A few members prepared drafts, which we read together and discussed. These written materials contained important analyses and allowed for the examination of different perspectives in regard to the same events. At the last meeting, in Israel in March 2019, we focused on how we would draw the group meetings to a close.

In what follows, I will share some observations that report my personal understanding of the group process. I will describe what I learned from my German colleagues. And I will make concluding remarks about how the group developed during 14 years of meetings. It is not my objective to suggest that there are answers to how and why the process unfolded as it did, only to lay it bare, from my point of view, in the hope that it can evoke new thinking about traumatic events and their transformation.

The Beginning

The project grew out of a casual meeting between Raimund Rumpeltes, a member of the German analytic group, and me at a conference in Warsaw in 2004. It took only a fleet of a moment to understand that our personal histories were intertwined in a mysterious way. It was not just the similar age and profession that connected us, but the unspoken intuition that we belong to opposite poles of the same catastrophe. And this was, I believe, what attracted us to each other. For me it was an opportunity to "peak in" on the demonized "other" that I have never met. I assumed that the same was true for him, meeting a Jewish person who is a second-generation survivor. In this enigmatic context, a year later, Raimund and I decided to create a German–Israeli psychoanalytic working group.

Before our first meeting in 2006, I had the following dream: *I was traveling with friends on a bus, and everything seemed fine except the fact that I was sleeping on a shelf in the overhead compartment* . . . . I understood that past and present merged in the context of the intensity of the upcoming meeting of the group. Sleeping on a shelf has a threatening connotation in our culture because of its resonance with situations in concentration camps.

During the first session, one Israeli member became nauseous and went out to vomit; we understood that it was a reaction to something that was indigestible in the room. Obviously, this "something" was the core issue of the project: to face that which is indigestible and yet transmitted from one generation to the next. On the next day, an Israeli analyst presented a case of a woman who had insisted on talking directly to the Germans in the group via a recording to share her memories from the Holocaust as well as her outrage. This had a devastating impact. The Germans felt accused, became defensive, and announced that they would not be able to participate in the project if they were to be blamed. For them, this was too much to contain. Complicated. I thought to myself: How could we steer clear of their feelings of guilt? In my mind, at that time, *they* definitely represented the perpetrators, and *we* were the victims.

As tensions eased, we began to share our complex histories. We asked ourselves, "Why are we here?" I told the group that my father had been engaged to a German whom he had to leave behind, which remains a missing link in his personal history and probably mine, too. During the next annual meeting, in Heidelberg, we were exposed to the crude realities of the past as a German analyst took out a dark leather album decorated by the German eagle on the cover. Inside were pictures of his Nazi relative that he presented to us directly. I was shocked by the realization that a member of our group was so closely connected to the Nazi past. At the same time, I was deeply moved by the courage of the German analyst to initiate acknowledgment of his past. This revelation evoked emotional turbulence in the group; the Germans did not know about their colleague's past. The Israelis were shocked.

The Process

There were several moments of dread. During our second visit to Heidelberg, a German member reported a dream: *a little black cat was put in an oven by mistake. The cat was half-scorched but still alive* . . . . As the group discussed the dream, images of crematoriums and burned bodies emerged. We wondered if our group was on fire, whether individually and collectively, we would be able to survive the dread that emerged so concretely in that moment.

On another occasion, while in Heidelberg, we went to a jazz concert in a nearby town. As we arrived at our destination, a small town known for its chemical factories, we were told that Cyclone B (the gas that was used in concentration camps to kill Jews and others) was manufactured there. We got out of the car; I sensed a strong smell of the chemicals and had a small anxiety attack. In this instance, the past was manifested in the present in powerfully threatening ways. Afterward, the Germans apologized and told us that they felt guilty for failing to foresee that this location may evoke a traumatic experience for us. Sadly, they explained that they are so accustomed to living side by side with these residuals of their past and that they hardly notice them. This event became a "now moment" in the group's history. It exposed the inner reality in which each of us exists: in a fleeting moment, the Israelis experienced past traumas in the present and revived deeply ingrained sensitivities. The Germans had to face their dissociated mode of experience and the shocking revelation of the way they had made themselves immune to the horrors of their pasts.

A presentation of a case by a German member also brought out ghosts from the closet. The analyst described the treatment hour, and the Israelis felt that she was inattentive to the patients' needs. There emerged a discussion about the patient's request to get another pillow and the analyst's refusal to provide it. The Israeli reaction became increasingly critical, even hostile, and was fused with prejudices and preconceptions about the Germans. Finally, we expressed our disagreement and criticism by suggesting that the presenter worked like a "Nazi analyst." This judgment was connected to the Kleinian inclinations of the analyst and the Israeli group's feeling that his strict approach reflected German meanness and rigidity. The

German analyst, almost in tears, left the room. We felt paralyzed and did not know how to resolve the situation. It was hard to think. There was a heavy silence. Only later could we reflect on the situation and connect it to the imprinted cultural differences and collective traumas that inform all of our differing perceptions. At the same time, we all appreciated the fact that now we were reacting freely to such differences, even fighting and not feeling the need to be defensive. This process provided a helpful repair and insight into our different patterns as analysts.

The written accounts that we created toward the end of the group meetings became a potential space for transformation and transcendence of such events. We could consider the event with less emotional involvement and more "professionally." We realized in the case of the "German analyst," as in other instances, that each group adheres to different psychoanalytic schools of thought and that this dissimilarity is in part derived from cultural differences. The Germans were oriented to Klein's theory. The Israelis in the group were more oriented to Kohutian and Winnicottian thinking, less drive theory and more contextual concepts.

As the group coalesced and became able to directly confront our differences, our reactions became more elaborated, and our associations developed further. For example, as a further elaboration on the event in which we criticized the German analyst, we touched on the issue of "cruelty" toward patients and soon found ourselves slipping again into stereotypes: are the Germans less empathic to their patients? Are they "colder?" Do they work rigidly by the book or by the law? Are the German clinical attitudes and approaches a function of their heritage? Many of the German analysts had been trained by analysts who had completed their training at former Nazi-connected institutes. Was the fascist culture imprinted in their professional attitudes? These questions were also raised, to our surprise, by German members who were concerned about whether the psychoanalytic tradition in Germany was influenced by Nazi ideology.

Over time, we touched on the link between the personal histories of our patients and our own historic cultural milieus from which we draw our understanding as analysts. We became more aware of the ways that historical events shape our lives, including our professional values. We recognized that history cannot be detached from our sense of self; we are born with our past and initially carry it with us into the future. At the same time, we assumed that we are free to choose whether to submit to our heritage or to transcend it and transform our preconceptions.

Sometimes, during our meetings, I had horrifying private associations. I remembered an uncle telling me about his childhood memories of the humiliation of Jews in Essen. Jews had to bend down and clean the streets with their beards. I have to assume that my mother must have witnessed that as a child. These thoughts emerged in my mind in confused and terrifying ways. Were these unconscious projections, or were they connected to a present, significant reality? I did not know.

My participation in the group for 14 years had a transformative impact on me. I became aware, more than ever before, of my grandfather, who was deported to Auschwitz. I knew that my mother had submitted a written statement to Yad Vashem, the Holocaust Museum in Jerusalem, in 1956, evidence that she knew what had happened to him. But this fact was never mentioned to me at home. Now, being refocused and newly motivated by our work in the group, I visited the memorial center in Paris to search for more information about my grandfather. I searched and found his name engraved on the wall. I also received an official document that specified the names of people who were in the convoy that took him to his final destination, Auschwitz. The document said (in French) that he had been "immediatement gasse" (instantly gassed).

What had been a missing link now became foremost in my mind, even comprehensible. Until then, my grandfather was a faceless person in my mind. I had not thought about him much. Now, Elias Kagan has become a person with his own subjectivity. I could think about him and imagine his life. I believe that the group contributed to this transformation, for which I am very grateful. This was part of the important reclaiming experience, uncovering the unspoken past and considering facts that had been hidden and even disavowed by our families. We could acknowledge the link between past, present, and future as an extension of our own continuity of being.

Even though we know that some parents spoke openly about their traumas, it seemed that many wished to spare their children from the traumas of the past. Yet, this pact of silence frequently evoked elaborate dreadful fantasies in the minds of the children of the second- and third-generation survivors.

I discovered that German families, too, had disguised facts about their parents, grandparents, and relatives. Silencing seemed to be a common experience, even if for very different reasons: in our Israeli families, dissociation functioned as protection from mental pain and survivor guilt. Sadness was disavowed, and fear was disguised while heroism, courage, and hope were cultivated in our upbringing. In the German families, silence was a function of shame, guilt, and a wish to deny what the parents did during the war. In all families, German and Israeli, traumatic events were often dealt with through a wish not to know too much about the past. In most families, there was a rupture in relational continuity across generations.

Eventually, we realized that we no longer needed "Group Separate." Mutual recognition and a sense of relative safety among the participants had slowly evolved, and we were able to forego the protective setting of the separate group. This turn of events was viewed favorably by all, and we were hopeful about our future.

In spite of the trust and optimism, new challenges came up. In particular, two wars in Gaza (in 2012 and 2014) raised questions about Israeli concern for the safety of peoples on its border. The Germans began to express interest in the Palestinian problem and visited Jenin, a Palestinian city in the West Bank. I thought that this was a sign of there being more freedom in the group to think and act in ways that might be critical of Israelis, freedom to disagree, and an evolution of potential space in the group. However, during the night of their visit to Jenin, the Germans were caught in the midst of a Molotov cocktail attack. Their hostel was on fire. They barely escaped. They came back worn out and shocked. The result was confusion. The political reality of the Middle East was violent, perplexing, and difficult to comprehend.

We Israelis had to face our own aggressive tendencies and deal with the politics of our government. Complex questions were raised by the Israeli members: What happened to the so-called Beautiful Israeli, the one characterized in local literature and the media during Israel's founding years by an enormous passion for building a haven/heaven for the Jewish people as well as a just society? How can we incorporate contradicting tendencies such as being children of refugees who lost everything, on the one hand, and being aggressors who, at times, become entangled in ethical dilemmas that seem to disavow our own past as refugees, on the other hand? These issues led the group to explore the lost potential in Israel and the possibility of its retrieval, "*re*membering" that which is *dis*membered and disavowed. We found ourselves in the unusual situation of discussing these issues among ourselves in the presence of Germans and with the Germans. Bringing these issues out into the open was an enriching experience. With the Germans, we experienced a compassionate search for a lost internal home of safety. Both Israelis and Germans felt longings for lost innocence in the most profound manner.

As the group aged and matured, one of the important experiences for me occurred in a meeting in which a discussion of social violence stirred up recollections of personal experiences: several members shared memories of being exposed to sexual or physical abuse at home. Others spoke about their parents' emotional blindness and lack of concern. No longer were we speaking of "Germans" vis-à-vis "Israelis." We understood that many of us were exposed to similar spates of parental aggression or social aggression tied to our traumatic past and that we all experienced radioactive identifications[2] (Gampel, 2000).

Such insights offered each of us an opportunity to broaden his or her perspective and allowed for shifts in the mind. At this latter stage in the group's history, our dialogue transcended splits: we could now more easily share experiences of vulnerability and pain. I not only expanded my awareness of my personal history but also learned about the traumas of the "others" and the profound anguish of those who were raised in ex-Nazi environments and continue to struggle with the manifestations of this background at present. The Germans could understand our anguish as citizens of a country that has lost some of its fundamental ideals. While clearly disavowing any moral or destructive equivalence between genocide in the Holocaust and Israeli aggression against Palestinians, we came to acknowledge that victims could turn out to be aggressors, and perpetrators could turn out to be victims and that those who are just at one point may become unjust at another point. We could appreciate the infinite changeability in our lives. We renounced fixed designations.

All the foregoing arose naturally in the group setting as nuanced reflections on our past and on the present. I experienced, as I believe all of us did, ups and downs, moments of deep friendship side by side with moments of disappointment and distrust, inclusion and exclusion, cohesion and fragmentation. We hosted each other in our homes, introduced our families, ate

2 Yolanda Gampel (2000) coined the concept "radioactive identification" to serve as a metaphoric representation of the violent penetration of social violence into the individual's psyche. The individual internalizes the radioactive remnants of which he is unaware of, and they destroy her from within. This can be manifested in various ways, from malignant identification with the aggressor or other symptoms. This identification is transmitted from one generation to the next.

meals together, walked together, and laughed together (many times about ourselves). We sometimes felt angry and alienated from each other.

Certainly, what started as a split between the "Germans" and the "Israelis" transformed into other kinds of split situations between leaders and non-leaders and between different psychoanalytic orientations. There was a vast range of experiences, many of which can be captured in writing and formulated now.

Analyzing Traumatic Internalizations: A Clinical Example

A short vignette will illustrate the kind of clinical materials that were used for our discussions. The example demonstrates the gradual evolution of memory and expansion of the mind in the analysis of an Israeli woman.

The patient is a successful professional, a ballet dancer, and has a fulfilling life with her husband and children. Soon after we met, she reported that her father was a detainee in Mengale's[3] clinic in Auschwitz. Since he died from heart disease when she was a child, she could not retrieve any details about his experiences in the camp. She felt that her mother refrained from discussing these experiences.

At the beginning of the analysis, she presented her first dream: *There is a dark object at the bottom of the sea. I can only observe it from above. It is untouchable.* We assumed that the dream related to the dreadful events of the Holocaust and mental pain that could not be touched yet.

In the third year of the analysis, the patient mentioned that she has a habit of grinding her teeth. In her associations, she recalled that Mengele gave her father a choice between having his teeth pulled out or being castrated. He chose to have his teeth pulled out. She realized that her habit of grinding her teeth has to do with a need to reassure herself that her teeth are intact. More so, she also realized that his choice actually permitted her to come to life.

The patient was very aware of mind–body connections. She felt that psychic trauma is transferred into the body when the mind cannot contain it.

3 Josef Mengale was a German SS officer and physician during World War II, notorious for his inhuman medical experiments on prisoners at Auschwitz concentration camp. Often referred to as the "Angel of Death," he conducted brutal experiments, particularly on twins and individuals with disabilities, in pursuit of his racial and genetic theories, and as such are considered examples of medical torture.

Therefore, it could not be "investigated" only verbally; she felt that she had to explore her own bodily sensations very attentively, as she did as a child when she was unable to communicate with her father verbally (he spoke only German, and she spoke only Hebrew. She believed that this situation was not accidental).

At some point, the patient decided to learn the German language. She felt that if she could speak "his" language, she may *transform the hidden barrier into a path of communication.* A few months later she and her husband decided to take a vacation in the Black Forest (*Schwartzwald*), a district in Germany which is known for its attractions for children. When she came back, she told me that the family had a great time. However, she was sick with a gum infection all week. She also reported two dreams that she had during this vacation: one was that *she had a taste of calcium oxide in her mouth. It was impossible to swallow it, disgusting and dreadful.* In the second dream, *she met with her father and asked all the questions that she always wanted to ask. With each question, he shrunk and became more nervous. She asked him to speak Yiddish. Suddenly, her mother appeared in the dream, and they hugged. Her dialogue with him was interrupted.* The patient said that there were many issues with "the mouth" during the vacation. She felt that it had to do with accumulated internalized aggression, having to shut up, refraining from expressing anger or screaming at her father, and being excluded from the parental discourse. She turned herself into a silent selfobject for her suffering father and accepted the formula that he was able to offer her as her father.

At the same time, we also considered her "bodily empathy" with her father: the symptom allowed her to intuit, via her body, the unspeakable sensations that her father could have had. The unknowable resided in the body and became a private shared space between the patient and the father. Understood this way, her suffering not only was projected onto her but resulted from her attempt to immerse herself in the absent father and decipher his mental state. A disposition of somatic interconnectedness was constituted so that she could intuit his disavowed pain.

She explained:

> The teeth were weak and broken due to the force that was put on them. . . . He whitewashed everything so that I would not speak to him, and more so, in order that he wouldn't ever need to talk to me. He chose my mother because she is so concrete and unable to touch.

And she continued:

> I, too, like to eat very hard food: the crust of the bread, green apples, and peel. I feel the connection between the gums and the heart,[4] the ear, nose and mouth. . . . During the week in Germany, I felt that my gums burned. My teeth grew from the injured gums. I ate only yogurt. . . . I wrote in my diary: My mother was connected to life from the outside, whereas I had to carry the death and the suffering from within. Six months later, she reported another dream: *My husband and I wanted to kiss. I took out the white chewing gum from my mouth. I was surprised that I could do that.*

Concluding Remarks

Reclaiming Unlived Experiences: Unthinkable Anxiety and Nameless Dread

The mind has mysterious ways of preserving dreadful experiences and can be captured by them. The self builds defensive mechanisms to protect itself through disavowal, dissociation, and splitting. Nonetheless, shadows of dread will inevitably return, not necessarily via direct experiencing but within dreams, reverie, visual images, and bodily sensations. Unthinkable anxiety and nameless dread are experienced in many ways and are transmitted from generation to generation. Children of parents who endured trauma are often unable to decipher their parents' state of mind. At the same time, they perceive the parent's vulnerability, their hidden longings for what was lost, and their fears of fragmentation.

The vignette exemplifies how unspoken dread was registered in the mind and body of a patient and assumed a singular form. Yet traumatic experiences and "radioactive" environments have infinite ways of registering in the mind. Within the Israeli–German group, we tried to touch on these experiences and share them. The group's consistent conviction to do the utmost to courageously engage with the past helped transform dissociated materials into thinkable events. There was a gradual expansion of the mind because of the group's members' willingness to surrender to the eye of the storm and experience it.

4 There is a known connection between gum disease and heart failure. Both illnesses can develop due to bacteria that are situated in the gum and later on in blood vessels that nurture the heart.

Vertical and Horizontal Splits

The reluctance to think about certain experiences, dissociate them, or hide them, signifies that such experiences are overly shame-engendering and too painful. A split is constituted to divide that which is thinkable from that which is unthinkable. Another form of split is found in the stereotyped convictions about "the Germans" or "the Israelis." We tend to automatically assume that what we know about them is correct. Our mind is preoccupied with accepted assumptions that block out new perspectives. Rigid attitudes stem from a reluctance to know the "other." Such attitudes cultivate self-cherishing and unmodified defensive grandiosity. This is a process of *ex*clusion rather than *in*clusion, which confines our mental and emotional freedom.

A wider perspective demands that prejudices be renounced as part of a quest for inner freedom, flexibility, concern for others, and transformation of the mind. The option to meet others' catastrophes can derive from the understanding that our core selfhood does not need to be caught up exclusively in our own identifications with our particular fate. The self can experience compassion and be open to a broad range of contextual events.

The enormous value of the unbiased state of the mind is recognized primarily in psychoanalytic thinking. We can refer to Kohut's (1966) concepts of "selfobjecting" and "transience," Bion's (1967) suggestion that we work "without memory, without desire and without understanding," and Winnicott's (1971, pp. 95–103, 1992, pp. 145–157) idea of potential space and the unintegrated position of the self. These mental states require an act of renunciation (Epstein, 2007). This concept, renunciation, refers to the ability to maintain an equanimous attitude in conflicting situations and not be attached to one perspective. In an open state of mind, one is more likely to be able to listen, accept complex situations, and decipher their meaning lucidly without collapsing into excessive emotional contaminations (Mann, 2020). The open position frees the mind from its tendency to attach unproductively to preconceived attitudes.

This act of renunciation occurred in our group during many good moments, when we could eliminate the glass wall that stood between preconceptions in regard to "us" and "them" and embrace the complexity of our situations and encounter an infinite interconnectedness of which we are part (Mann, 2013, 2015). In these moments, we experienced a sort of twinship (Togashi, 2014), mutual empathy (Pillsbury, 2019), and a sense of entanglement as professional colleagues and friends. We shared our own impermanence, getting older within these 14 years, and we could feel its impact. We could experience the profound significance of "being human among humans" (Kohut, 1984, p. 200).

Can the Self Free Itself From Its Own Traumas?

The distinctive characteristic of the group was that its members were committed to analyzing the constraining influence of trauma. We understood that we could respond genuinely and authentically to events in our lives only if we were able to recognize our embeddedness in and transferences to past traumatic experiences. We came to appreciate in a new way that we can open up a space for unmasking events that have engulfed us and carried us along in their wake. We proved to ourselves that by identifying repetitions, we can free ourselves, if only partially, from re-creating the circumstances that shaped our past.

But there is more to it. Freedom of the self is not just renunciation of our personal attachments to past traumas and learning from experience. "Full freedom" of the self would be attained if the self could fully disengage from its particular identities. Yet this is an unrealizable ideal situation. The mind cannot fully be freed or purified due to the depth of traumatic imprinting; we always remain with something incomprehensible and untransformable.

Seen this way, the decision to terminate was not a sigh of despair or exhaustion. We felt that we did what could be done. The group situation contributed greatly to transforming the trauma from a private disaster to a shared experience. Members of the group now have a better understanding of the traumas of the others. This is not to say that the group process eliminates personal traumas. Rather, it enhanced empathy and allowed us to perceive trauma as a collective catastrophe within a larger context. Our traumas gained significance that goes beyond the individual "me."

Each of us remained, I believe, with a meaningful experience and a sense of responsibility to carry on with transformation. For instance, one member of the group decided that he would work on global warming issues. Raimund Rumpeltes and I decided to create a new Israeli–German group of younger analysts. In this new group, we plan to make more consideration of cultural factors in remembering trauma and focusing more on the concerns of the younger generation. For the younger generation, the Holocaust may have less personal impact, but for them, it is likely to be highly relevant for thinking about potential future mass disasters. Both these instances reflect the effects of the group's cultivation of a perspective that goes beyond individual concerns and self-focused disasters to concerns for the human condition. It is a process of liberating the self from its own shadows.

References

Bion, W. R. (1967). Notes on memory and desire. *The Psychoanalytic Forum*, *2*, 272–273, 279–280.

Epstein, M. (2007). *Psychotherapy without the self: A Buddhist perspective*. Yale University Press.

Gampel, Y. (2000). Reflections on the prevalence of the uncanny in social violence. In A. C. G. M. Robben & M. M. Suárez-Orozco (Eds.), *Cultures under siege: Collective violence and trauma* (pp. 48–69). Cambridge University Press. http://catdir.loc.gov/catdir/samples/cam032/99049062.html

Kohut, H. (1966). Forms and transformations of narcissism. *Journal of the American Psychoanalytic Association*, *14*(2), 243–272.

Kohut, H. (1984). *How does analysis cure*? (A. Goldberg & P. Stepansky, Eds.). University of Chicago Press.

Mann, G. (2013). Being human among humans: Response to Maxwell S. Sucharov's "Thoughts on wholeness, connection, and healing: Moving toward complexity in the analytic space". *International Journal of Psychoanalytic Self Psychology*, *8*(4), 398–411. https://doi.org/10.1080/15551024.2013.825946

Mann, G. (2015). Paradoxes of belonging. *International Journal of Psychoanalytic Self Psychology*, *10*(3), 275–286. https://doi.org/10.1080/15551024.2015.1043844

Mann, G. (2020). Emptiness, equanimity and the selfobject function. *Psychoanalytic Inquiry*, *40*(5), 300–310. https://doi.org/10.1080/07351690.2020.1766321

Ornstein, A. (2004). *My mother's eyes Holocaust memories of a young girl*. Emmis Books.

Pillsbury, S. H. (2019). Mutual empathy: Imagined symbol and realization in the treatment of trauma. *Psychoanalysis, Self and Context*, *14*(3), 247–255. https://doi.org/10.1080/24720038.2019.1602135

Togashi, K. (2014). A sense of "being human" and twinship experience. *International Journal of Psychoanalytic Self Psychology*, *9*(4), 265–281. https://doi.org/10.1080/15551024.2014.947676

Winnicott, D. W. (1971). *Playing and reality*. Basic Books.

Winnicott, D. W. (1992). *Through paediatrics to psycho-analysis: Collected papers*. Karnac Books.

Chapter 5

"If You Don't See Me, I Will Show You"

The Paradox of Love in Therapy*

Introduction

In his 1912 paper, "On the Dynamics of Transference," Freud (1958a) suggests that:

> It must be understood that each individual, through the combined operation of his innate disposition and the influences brought to bear on him during his early years, has acquired a specific method of his own in his conduct of his erotic life – that is, in the preconditions to falling in love which he lays down, in the instincts he satisfies and the aims he sets himself in the course of it. This produces what might be described as a stereotype plate (or several such), which is constantly repeated – constantly reprinted afresh – in the course of the person's life . . . If someone's need for love is not entirely satisfied by reality, he is bound to approach every new person whom he meets.
>
> (pp. 99–100)

In other words, an unsatisfied need for love evolves into a constant search for it. This pursuit, of course, also reaches the therapist. Thus, the patient's love for the therapist is a significant cornerstone oiling the wheels of the psychoanalytic process. According to Freud, the love of a patient is always a derivative of sexuality, even if it appears to be pure and devoid of sensuality. It may lead to a breakthrough and to the opening up of muted areas of the psyche. However, it may also lead to resistance and to a negative tendency when touching upon conflictual aspects that divert the treatment from its real objective.

* This chapter is based on Mann (2014).

DOI: 10.4324/9781003449386-5

Due to these risks, which lie in wait for the therapist, Freud suggests that the analyst be especially cautious, pointing to the great value of a restrained approach. In "Recommendations to Physicians Practicing Psycho-Analysis" (first published in 1912), Freud (1958b) wrote:

> I cannot advise my colleagues too urgently to model themselves during psycho-analytic treatment on the surgeon, who puts aside all his feelings, even his human sympathy, and concentrates his mental forces on the single aim of performing the operation as skillfully as possible. . . . He (the patient) would like to reverse the situation, and finds the analysis of the doctor more interesting than in his own. . . . The doctor should be opaque to his patients and, like a mirror, should show them nothing but what is shown to him.
>
> (p. 115)

In his 1915 article "Observation on Transference-Love," Freud (1958c) noted how the mere experiment of letting oneself slide into affectionate feelings for the patient is not altogether without danger. After all, our control over ourselves is not so complete that we may not suddenly one time go beyond what we intended. However, Freud's conduct vis-à-vis his patients reveals that despite clear warnings, he himself was not immune to loving the patient. In fact, it is known that he spent time with his patients, sometimes taking care of funding their therapy, walking with some of them in the park, and even going on holiday with his patient, Sandor Ferenczi (Gay, 1988). After this incident, Freud admitted that this trip was a sign of his weakness. He himself was unable to control his countertransference and relate to Ferenczi in a sufficiently "analytic" manner in the way he did toward others, because he loved him too much.

Freud's decisive requirement began to change significantly from the 1950s onwards, when countertransference in general and feelings of love between the therapist and the patient in particular were seen more and more as a common field of experience, a place for the reconstruction of repetitious modes of contact as well as a potential ground for new experiences that did not exist in the original field in which the patient lived in the past.

In this regard, Winnicott, Kohut, and Ghent were the most prominent pioneers of the contextual approach. When Winnicott famously asserted that "there is no such thing as a baby" without there being maternal care, he clearly stated that the infant constitutes the mother as much as the mother constitutes the infant. Ostensibly, we see two individuals. In fact, however, one cannot exist without the other; we see a unity. So Winnicott creates a tapestry of inseparability. The mother is the infant's environment, and in this sense, she is the one who determines the direction of his development and, subsequently, his ability to use her.

In 1967, Winnicott expanded the contextual emphasis when he published "The Mirror-Role of Mother and Family in Child Development" (Winnicott, 2016, pp. 211–218). What was initially Freud's neutral mirror has now become life-giving, creating a mirror of the self and his being. The mother observes the baby, and her facial fluctuations indicate that she sees him. If so, her face is the precursor of the mirror. The girl who will one day look in the mirror will see in it what she saw in her mother's eyes. She will see herself as her mother once saw her, her mother's affirming look. She will then know that she exists and will have the capacity to look into herself. It is important to emphasize the subjective – rather than the objective – reflection as a central pillar in comprehending the function of the mirror.

On the other hand, when the mother's face is impenetrable, what the infant sees is the mother's mood or her rigid defenses. Here, the mirror is opaque, and the baby's creative ability is lost while desperately searching for something in the environment that will provide her with a more explicit answer. This search for a substitute for the mirror function fills the place of what could have been a quiet and fruitful interaction with the surrounding world. What is important in this context is the extent to which it is possible or impossible to anticipate the mother's face. The absence of the ability to predict her response leads to chaos in the infant's world. He will never know what to expect and will therefore look around insecurely. The opaque sight becomes something to look at, rather than something to look into and be immersed with, an objective object rather than a subjective object. In such a situation, men fall in love with beauty instead of loving a girl and finding out what is beautiful about her. In other words, the mode of mirroring becomes crucially important. Genuine mirroring works to constitute a true self. An opaque mirroring leads to the constitution of a false self.

Winnicott developed such contextual thinking while he already viewed therapy as playing within a boundless potential space with infinite possible happenings. Psychoanalytic therapy is the sandbox of therapists and patients, where it is possible to be immersed in the patient's subjective reality as long as one adheres to the fundamental rules of the game; one never strives to check the objective credibility or the realization of the experience in reality. In the introduction to *Playing and Reality* (1971, p. xxi), Winnicott wrote, "My contribution is to ask for a paradox to be accepted and tolerated and respected, and for it not to be resolved." This is the paradox of playing and reality.

In Winnicott's conceptual thinking, the way to reality always passed via an illusion. It is only fitting that certain wishes can exist in the transitional space of the experience: I am allowed to be the infant who exists within the adult; I am permitted to be the adult who exists in the infant; I am permitted to ask to be an object of desire; I am allowed to disclose my most hidden wishes; I am entitled to lack common sense, to be devoid of any rationality. I am allowed! In this sense, the analysis is a playground of desires and needs. The therapeutic encounter facilitates these possibilities. It is here that the self-yearning to be loved receives the full inspiration for as long as necessary until one day, her selfhood will be constituted, even in the absence of the therapist's love.

It is important to bear in mind that so long as desires exist as wishes, they maintain the transitional quality as an arena of play. Their realization overturns the rules of the game and destroys the illusion's curative capacity. Furthermore, the process cannot be circumvented or shortened. The patient's self needs the possibility of immersing itself in such yearnings, of using the language of desire or need, and of imagining their representations. It is appropriate that he be able to use these contents as material in the hands of its creator.

There Is a Process in the Paradox

The patient's love of the therapist may be based on a yearning that the therapist will provide an infinite space for tenderness, be a "life giver" (Symington, 1993), a "transformational object" (Bollas, 1987), or a selfobject (Kohut, 1984) that fulfills these functions and provides a possibility to expand the patient's experiences and needs.

During an analytical session, a patient recounted the following:

What do I feel as I lie on the couch? I feel what I have fantasized about for years, being like a child at home,
Who lies on a bed in the room,

And everything around is quiet, tranquil, and green.
Had I covered myself with a blanket, I really wouldn't have been able to get up from there.
So foolish . . .
I cry.
Now.
After all, I truly gave up this phantasy so long ago,
And I don't miss it.
Because I don't need it with them.
And since you courageously created this place for me,
And make it so simple and so available; perhaps now I can be loved?
Perhaps I can even dare to love?
I am anxious,
To return to this previous place . . .
If, for some reason which I won't understand, you reject me,
If you won't love me,
I will still be a patient,
but without this feeling of endless support.
You are the first person who made me feel that I'm not alone . . .
that is why you appeared in my dreams.
and that is why I stayed here for so long.

These words illustrate a place in which the therapy promotes vitality and an experience of self-worth. The validated patient feels that there is a "home" in the presence of the therapist. With adequate mirroring, the patient's narcissistic needs are met, and he senses the possibility of feeling loved and perhaps even of loving others. He says quite openly that he wants to "be completely loved." This need was denied by him for many years.

This kind of revitalization occurs in transformational moments, "now moments," (Stern et al., 1998) or "aesthetic" moments (Bollas, 1987) that cultivate renewed hope. A restrained experience of intimacy may emerge, perhaps accompanied by tranquil sexuality. With reference to Freud's work on transference, Takeo Doi (1973), a Japanese analyst explains that transference is linked to non-verbal dependence and reliance on others. Such dependence, which he terms the psychology of "Amea," exists between children and their parents, as well as between young and elder people. It is a model of human relations with no need to verbalize it. Doi, like Ghent (1990), suggests that the need to be dependent is universal. It is a nonsexual search for closeness and connectedness. Accepting this yearning without interpretation removes the tension and guilt from it.

The therapist, who functions as a selfobject, allays the patient's dread of closeness and fear of love, stemming from the fear of re-traumatization and past experiences of vulnerability. The patient feels understood. In fact, a central aspect of his need has been met. There is no longer a need for sexualization.

Glenn Gabbard, a psychologist who deals with ethical issues in therapeutic situations, demonstrates a different set of circumstances when describing his sessions with a patient named Barbara.[1] He describes the following situation:

> A patient arrived who felt that she was going nowhere in her life and was uncertain about who she really was. At a certain stage of the treatment Barbara felt disappointed by her fiancé's capacity to pay her the "loving attention" that she longed for. It was then that the first signs of erotic attachment to the therapist appeared in the therapy. The fiancé was "incredibly jealous," and Barbara loved it because "it made him worry" about her. She explained that jealousy makes him more attentive.

Barbara sensed Gabbard's nonresponsiveness and then intensified her efforts to attract him, this time by the way she dressed. She now also wanted to know "[a]ll about him." Gabbard comments: "It sounds like you want to figure out exactly what I'm like, so you can adapt yourself to my preferences." Barbara confirms that that is what she has always done with men and continues to demand that Gabbard tell her everything about himself, whether he is married or how old he is. Gabbard wondered why these facts were so important to her.

She then intensified the pressure to see beads of sweat on his face. Perhaps she should come to the session dressed in especially sexy underwear? In the same breath, she said:

> You know, sexuality is actually quite foreign to me . . . . I don't flirt . . . . It doesn't come naturally to me. I use sex to compensate for *not* feeling that I am really a hot shot.

1 This section is based on Gabbard (2009).

This dialogue between patient and therapist clearly shows that Barbara's courting of Gabbard did not stem from sexual urges alone. The sexualization of the relationship was intended to compensate for the lack of self-esteem and was linked more to a humiliating need to satisfy the other. This is an example of a situation in which a profound need to be noticed takes a perverse turn when the relationship doesn't provide a response to the mirroring and idealization needs of the patient. The absence of any resonance whatsoever only reinforced the patient's entreaty: "I have to sleep with you so that I can feel sufficiently worthwhile."

I believe that in such a situation, where the patient's neediness becomes so evident, one can offer her a response that is more "personal" so that she would feel more understood. For example, it would have been possible to respond to one of her "personal" questions. In my view, one can hear such questions as a sincere and profound appeal to the therapist, a wish to know if he is sufficiently well versed in the complexities of relationships or whether he is of an appropriate age to be a protective parent. I listen to the transferential quality of the questions and the meaning enfolded within them and respond in a measured and fitting way without even interpreting them. I wish to encourage the patient to ask, to investigate, to raise the questions that preoccupy him and not act to silence him.

A certain responsiveness prevents reconstructing self-humiliation and so sets in motion the capacity to create a different relationship with another, in which mutual respect and mutual regulation determine the process. We try not to encourage repetitions of past pathology but to cocreate a new experience (Lachmann & Beebe, 1996). A stance such as this by the therapist avoids the patient's need to continually slide – even within the therapeutic hour – into the degrading and perverted areas of supplication, which were her lot for so many years, to beg for human contact. An empathic stance calms the sexualization in the transference and facilitates a transformation, first in the mind of the therapist (Symington, 2007) and subsequently in the mind of the patient. This makes it possible to reactivate and to reinforce the playful, creative potential of the patient.

It is important to emphasize that tranquil sexuality turns into paradox-breaking sexualization when it becomes the sole means of achieving an objective and not just yet another experience within the numerous experiences of the self in the analytic process. Sexualization aimed at a singular objective narrows the range of self-experiences.

In various writings, Gabbard (1994, 2003) deals with the therapist's anxiety and tension in light of his patient's yearning for erotic impulsivity. In such situations, the way in which this tension is held in the therapist's mind is highly significant. Therapists sometimes find it difficult to cope with their patients' erotic yearnings. If so, the option of avoiding the area of temptation becomes especially attractive. Gabbard (2003) admits that he was discomforted by his patient's open confession of love for him. Gabbard describes how he sat behind the couch and felt uneasy. He thought about his own anxiety and realized that the expression of love toward him made him uncomfortable. He hurriedly changed the subject to what had happened between the patient and his father. He directed the patient to talk about the past rather than the present.

At the same time, Gabbard also reminds us that excitation in the therapeutic relationship may serve not only the patient but also the therapist. This possible direction occurs when the therapist is, in fact, himself in a situation of narcissistic disequilibrium due to his own personal issues. In this situation, fanning the flame of eroticism and abandoning his function as the bearer of the patient's suffering serves the therapist's narcissistic needs. Consequently, instead of the therapist being a selfobject for the patient, it is the patient who actually fulfills that function for the therapist.

However, when the therapist has the capacity to create a tranquil and sufficiently free zone within his mind, he can identify the deep roots of his vulnerability and his needs and transform excitation into empathy, recognizing the line between regressive desire and tranquil love. How is that transformation in the therapist's mind to be explained?

Transformations of the mind require patience and courage. For instance, being aware of an erotic fantasy without pushing it aside, allowing an overwhelming pleasant feeling or one which is unpleasant to sink in and be, letting the process come into being without refusal, and being willing to "bear" it. As the process continues, the therapist may realize the enriching potential and the hope that is enfolded in the patient's desperate search for love. The therapist will comprehend that the patient tries to communicate his needs with a stammer, the only way available to him, perhaps due to a feeling that he won't be heard if he isn't sufficiently blunt or possibly as a repetitive use of his archaic objects' language. The therapist may pick up a communication: What is missing here in this process? What does the patient need? These questions are materials that can be thought about and deciphered together with the patient. The therapist can share his reflections with the patient, wonder whether sexualization is a defensive response to an empathic failure, and provide a response to the unvocalized need. Thus, the patient can feel that he is being treated in an open, respectful, and transformative manner.

These are reflections that may lead to a transformation toward compassion in the mind of the therapist. He will not limit himself to interpretations that relate to resistance, such as "the patient is now acting out" or "attacking the therapy." It is important that the therapist be in subtle connection with the patient's momentary delicate emotional vicissitudes and attempt to sense their profound essence. The immediate appearance does not reveal their entire significance; what seems to be driven by sexuality is not always derived from that particular urge. By means of prolonged immersion that suspends interpretation, a connection to the deeper narcissistic motives becomes possible. We are reminded of Winnicott's (1971) paradox of *Playing and Reality*, as mentioned before.

Children claim that "when you break the rules, you don't get to play anymore." And indeed, when quiet sexuality is replaced by realized sexualization, the play is over. No longer is there a paradox. Everything has turned into reality.

What appears to be surrender becomes submission. Ghent (1990) describes surrender and submission and places one against the other as two experiences that are seemingly alike but are essentially different. Surrender stems from a profound readiness to be handed to the "other." It lacks any dimension of control, inspection, or demandingness. It is derived from the area of faith (Eigen, 1981). It is a capacity to shed the defenses of the false self by a belief in a present other, perhaps even a wish to be known to him and to know him. On the other hand, submission is nothing more than a deceptive disguise for a violent negation of the true self in the name of the untrustworthy allure of the other's support. In an environment of continuous impasse, submission develops in the hope that there will eventually be a new beginning as a solution to the previous fragmentation of the self. The positive needs, to be known and to know the other, are converted into consent to be penetrated and invaded by him, provided that his presence is maintained.

In the therapeutic dialogue, the propensity toward submission can develop as a transferential event. The patient – lacking confidence in the therapist as a benevolent object – is liable to search for a way to develop an erotic connection to the therapist so long as she doesn't cease to impress him or perhaps in order not to lose him. Here the consent to submission is a kind of imposed solution in the struggle against solitude and in an attempt not to remain without a contextual matrix. Though the patient doesn't remain alone, her core self remains isolated, split and prevented from developing its own cohesiveness.

A patient once said to me: "If I am not being seen, then I'll show them." This sentence contains everything that happened on those occasions that repeated themselves again and again when she, as a baby, as a child, and as a woman, searched for approval from her mother, her surroundings, and her partner. When these didn't come in a timely manner, she resorted to more invasive tendencies to enlist the validation she considered essential for her existence by indulging in false relations and constituting false mirroring. The potential of having innocent relations of intimacy and love easily gives way to substitutes at times of distress. Disappointment of being seen by beneficent eyes leads more than once to provocative activities, perhaps in a way similar to Barbara's actions. Then, instead of being seen, she acts in a way that will ensure that she *is* seen.

Another patient tells of her first meeting with her previous therapist:

> He waited for me outside to make it easier for me to find him or possibly to protect me from the frightening dogs that barked loudly as I approached. "Get used to it," he said as he extended a manly handshake. "They are not really as dangerous as they seem." Signs I did not know how to decipher . . .
>
> The first two years were somewhat of a blur. Conversations about childhood, mother, work, here and there. I developed a sensitive ear. I knew how to talk in an enchanting way. Above all, I knew what *not* to talk about: not about father, not about my husband and especially not about him. . . . He got under my skin, penetrated deeply into my soul. I began to live from one meeting to another, yearning for time off to stare into space, to fantasize and reconstruct every word. At the same time, he began to lose weight and to dress up like a peacock (at the time I didn't know that he was in the process of parting from his wife). I said to myself: "Here is the proof; it is real." I became mute. I didn't speak and he didn't ask. I began to construct shared dreams; how we would travel to the east, he would be the guide, I the companion. . . . The situation became insufferable, an obsession as if engraved in my flesh with no protective skin. I informed him that I wanted to end the treatment. He wasn't happy, yet another proof that he was "there." On the day we

parted, we hugged. . . . Tall but disappointing, not close, not fatherly, not friendly, not intimate.

But a good smell.

One holiday eve, the phone rings. "Happy holiday, how are you?" The stomach churned. I suggest a meeting. Not in the clinic but in a café.

In the first five minutes, I realized it was a terrible mistake. He wasn't there, a stranger, confused, helpless. I wanted the earth to devour me; I felt so humiliated, so small and so stupid.

Three years later, the phone rings again. This time he offers to refer a patient. Again, a cup of coffee. Talk about a patient. I tried to talk. . . . He did not remember. He did not know. Was he sorry if he had upset me?

We are here now, right? Come let us talk about the present.

The writing is on the wall, but I am blind. The same familiar feeling, a churning stomach.

Voices of reality circulate within me. For example, I ask myself: "What are you looking for"? Then, he begins to act: seduction, wooing, poems; focused on his target. . . .

The phantasy had been realized. At some moments, I felt like a queen, and everything else in life became insignificant. . . . I lied to the children, distanced myself from my friends and, in particular, from those who didn't buy into the rosy cloud, which I was then offering as an explanation. My husband was felt to be a shadow in the background. Life became increasingly reduced.

In other, more distant circles, I heard voices that praised the courage, the ability to go with what was really in my heart. Yet my voice, in the medley of these external voices and trapped from within, disappeared. When I tried to breathe in, as one does after a prolonged dive, a kind of doubt crept into my mind. Immediately, the opposing voice appeared, telling me that since he really knows me, since he is familiar with my veined fears, anxieties, and yearnings and still, nonetheless, chooses me,

Perhaps I am really worth it? But no, I wasn't worth it. I was a slave. Attentive to his needs, negating myself, erasing every feeling of pain.

Repressing the parting from my partner, my family. Crushing my former life into thin dust and sustained by the illusion: "Between us, there is something else."

But there was no love here; he made no commitment; he didn't deceive. It was only me who wanted it, and he was there in his own free zone, which belonged only to him.

> And if I just once dared to be less available, to hold on to something that was "mine," on the following day, he told me that he had been with another woman. I thanked him that he had left, that he had taken advantage of my family holiday to be with another woman and stay with her.
>
> I remained pained, helpless, filled with a sense of emptiness. Something inside me had been killed.
>
> Time passed.
>
> Somehow, I managed to emerge out of dense clouds of alcohol and to save myself. I dared to go back to therapy, this time, of course, to a female therapist, and most of the time, I have myself . . . and her.
>
> But sometimes it still comes back, feelings of shame and guilt, intense pain, a dreadful emptiness. How did I get there? What led me to deposit my soul like that? To submit? The memory is suffocating, and the guilt is overwhelming.

The patient told me her story, and I felt the piercing pain. I was amazed by the extent to which the experience was still ingrained in her psyche as well as in her body despite the lapse of time. I suggested that this relationship of just a few months, during which she had left her home, is connected to exploitation.

It was surprising that the patient denied my definition. She believed that these events did not stem in any particular way from exploitation but rather exposed a long-standing wound due to prolonged deprivation. As such, the pain only becomes more profound. The previous sense of lack, the loneliness, the absence of adequate responsiveness to her needs, all these feelings surfaced in a surprisingly precise way in the transference to her previous therapist.

It needs to be mentioned that the patient was the daughter of a mentally damaged Holocaust survivor. (Apparently, the mother had suffered sexual abuse in the woods in which she had been hiding with the partisans from the Nazis.) Throughout her childhood, the patient experienced her mother's psychic deadness. At the time of the previous therapy, she knew that there was a sexual attraction in the room and felt that the therapist desired her. She, however, continued to talk only about other matters. The attraction was never mentioned in the course of two years of therapy. She explained that this doesn't need to be seen as surprising; after all, she had never been able to talk about her needs or relate to them in any way. Any such talk only served to heighten the sense of shame and to serve as additional proof of her insufficiency. She had to protect a certain image of being jovial and smiling so as not to spoil the experience of having succeeded in impressing and attracting the therapist, the bearer of her lost grandiosity. Apparently, much like an ancient echo, her intuition signaled that if she were to talk about what she was feeling, she would destroy herself as well as the therapy in which she was invested. In the final analysis, she – not he – would have to carry the cross of her "destructive aggression" and her unbearable shame.

Thus, the impossibility of quiet sexuality and safe devotion paved the way for a masochist submission to these relations with him. For the patient, the wretched outcome was twofold: both a failure to transform her abiding suffering and a missed opportunity to be found and to be loved as she was and as she deserved to be.

Recognition of the patient's narcissistic needs, genuine mirroring and admiring – while the therapist remained resolute, his non-vindictiveness, his refusal to withdraw or become seductive – could have anchored the patient's needs in the reality of her therapy and integrated them inside an authentic self that lives and presents his subjective experiences joyfully without the need to hide. A therapist who allows a patient to make use of him in such a way and enables her to unfurl her needs while at the same time validating them by means other than satisfying those needs sets in motion a process of restoring the live self, the self that dares to expose an entire range of its needs and those concealed in his heart in the hope that there is an appropriate response to them.

However, in the absence of selfobject provision, the unmet narcissistic needs intensify and become a regressive force with an obsessive quality. Emmanuel Ghent (2001) distinguishes between "need" and "neediness." Whereas the first is a healthy narcissistic position, which Ghent describes as "watering newly planted flowers," the second, neediness, is evidence of a regression to a bygone state, an action that he describes as "weeding." Ghent suggests not to repeatedly focus on the "old" and reconstruction as it appears in transferential material. He draws attention to the importance of cultivating new experiences that promote hope and progression.

In the present context, neediness becomes apparent through relentless demandingness to realize love in therapy. Sexualization of this nature masks a real need for closeness and intimacy. It is a manifestation of the rupture of the self. Repetitive sexual longings indicate a split of the two axes (the narcissistic axis and the drive) and the latter taking over the narcissistic matrix

(Kohut, 2009).[2] The damaged self is unable to reorganize itself cohesively because the pull of regression is so powerful. The self protects itself from experiences of pain and narcissistic vulnerability when it converts feelings of anxiety, loneliness, and alienation into erotic fantasies that will serve as a substitute for the mirror function. This phenomenon, defined as "narcissistic desire" (Wolf, 1994), consists of an attempt to force the other to love the self. There is no tender love of object in such incidents but rather a compulsive love, with a quality of childish grandiosity, which creates a perverse solution for the damaged self.

This situation occurs when the selfobject fails to function, like those parents of Freud's hysterical patients who did not have the ability to respond to their children, improve, accept, and admire them when confronted by their Oedipal desires.

In a correct therapeutic context in which the therapist is not fearful, does not prevent the patient from divulging her most intimate wishes, and makes no attempt to realize those desires, sexualization regains its appropriate place in the narcissistic matrix. Tranquil sexuality and the initiation of authentic needs become possible. Neediness once more becomes the need. From this perspective, the disintegration that occurred in the transference may be a window of opportunity for the restoration of the self.

Closing Remarks

In this chapter, I have discussed the difference between tranquil sexuality and sexualization in therapy. The fluctuations between these two states are contextual. Tranquil sexuality facilitates the exploration of overt and hidden narcissistic needs within the course of the therapeutic process, while sexualization distorts narcissistic needs and promotes regressive behavior.

The last example I offered is taken from the analysis of a woman who experienced the malignant regression I described in connection to her

2 In his book *The Restoration of the Self* (2009), Kohut writes

> The infantile sexual drive in isolation is not the primary psychological configuration . . . The primary psychological configuration (of which the drive is only a constituent) is the experience of the relation between the self and the empathic self-object. . . . Drive manifestations in isolation establish themselves only after traumatic and/or prolonged failures in empathy from the side of the self-object environment. . . . If the self is seriously damaged, however, or destroyed, then the drives become powerful constellations in their own right. In order to escape from depression, the child turns from the unempathic or absent self-object to oral, anal, and phallic sensations, which he experiences with great intensity. (p. 122)

previous therapist. When she heard that I was going to discuss a paper by Glen Gabbard (2009) as part of a conference on the ethics of therapists, she asked if I would present her case. I agreed to use it in my discussion provided that *she* write it in her language, and *I* would read her text as written by her. This is the text I presented.

This responsiveness may be viewed as a non-verbal interpretation by way of an action. Sometimes, taking a stand – and more importantly, *how* we do so – is no less significant than a thousand explanatory words. I consider my agreeing to her request as a clear recognition of the wrong done to her and a validation of the distress that requires correction. For her, this act made it possible to close a circle, a possibility to transform the shame, the disgrace, and the narcissistic injury into an act of courage, assertiveness, and mature narcissism.

Furthermore, the opportunity to write her story as part of a conference on ethics made it possible to recall the emotional subtleties she had experienced at the time, to look in the mirror, and renovate the self-image of humiliation, turning it into an image of self-worth. Through a creative–aesthetic act, she could, at this point, write what should have been written a long time ago, not as an indictment but as a manifesto of professional ethics. This writing is akin to a dialogue between the fragmented self of that period and the restored self that understands what the right ideals are and is determined to realize them. Writing is an act of creativity. It promotes the transformation of archaic narcissism into mature narcissism.

Of course, the therapist's response to her request also conveyed to her that she was not "alone" in the process of healing this wound and that we were treating it together, producing a "shared" text that seats the two of us in one place. Contrary to past experiences, this time, the therapist gave her full trust, relied on her, and provided cover for the trust the patient placed in her.

On this note, we will return to the place where this chapter began, with the Freud of 1915. Freud (1958c) described a state of erotic infatuation that required realization. He suggested that the basis of this requirement was sexual, an unresolved Oedipal complex. Perhaps we can see in Freud's fascinating writings an inspiration for a broader observation, one that includes the context in which the patient eventually matured and not only sexuality. We will see the language of need and not just the language of desire. We will reach the realization that the need to be loved in therapy seems to be based on narcissistic needs that are not only sexual but often misidentified as such.

References

Bollas, C. (1987). *The shadow of the object: Psychoanalysis of the unthought known*. Columbia University Press.
Doi, T. (1973). *The anatomy of dependence*. Kodansha International.
Eigen, M. (1981). The area of faith in Winnicott, Lacan and Bion. *The International Journal of Psychoanalysis*, *62*(4), 413–433.
Freud, S. (1958a). The dynamics of transference. In J. Strachey & A. Freud (Eds.), *The standard edition of the complete psychological works of Sigmund Freud: Vol. 12 (1911–1913): The case of schreber papers on technique & other works* (pp. 97–108). Hogarth Press.
Freud, S. (1958b). Recommendations to physicians practicing psycho-analysis. In J. Strachley & A. Freud (Eds.), *The standard edition of the complete psychological works of Sigmund Freud: Vol. 12 (1911–1913): The case of schreber papers on technique & other works* (pp. 109–120). Hogarth Press.
Freud, S. (1958c). Observation on transference-love. In J. Strachley & A. Freud (Eds.), *The standard edition of the complete psychological works of Sigmund Freud: Vol. 12 (1911–1913): The case of schreber papers on technique & other works* (pp. 159–171). Hogarth Press.
Gabbard, G. O. (1994). On love and lust in erotic transference. *Journal of the American Psychoanalytic Association*, *42*(2), 385–403. https://doi.org/10.1177/000306519404200203
Gabbard, G. O. (2003). Miscarriages of psychoanalytic treatment with suicidal patients. *The International Journal of Psycho-Analysis*, *84*(Pt 2), 249–261. https://doi.org/10.1516/002075703321632720
Gabbard, G. O. (2009, March). *Erotic impasse in psychoanalytic treatment*. Lecture at Tel Aviv University's Psychotherapy Conference, Erotic Transference: A Breakthrough or Crossing a Border? Tel Aviv, Israel.
Gay, P. (1988). *Freud: A life for our time* (1st ed.). W.W. Norton & Company.
Ghent, E. (1990). Masochism, submission, surrender: Masochism as a perversion of surrender. *Contemporary Psychoanalysis*, *26*, 108–136. https://doi.org/10.1080/00107530.1990.10746643
Ghent, E. (2001). Need, paradox, and surrender: Commentary on paper by Adam Phillips. *Psychoanalytic Dialogues*, *11*(1), 23–41. https://doi.org/10.1080/10481881109348595
Kohut, H. (1984). *How does analysis cure?* University of Chicago Press.
Kohut, H. (2009). *The restoration of the self*. The University of Chicago Press.
Lachmann, F., & Beebe, B. (1996). The contribution of self and mutual regulation to therapeutic action: A case illustration. *Progress in Self Psychology*, *12*, 123–140.
Mann, G. (2014). If you don't see me, I will show you. *The Israeli Journal of Psychotherapy "Sihot"*, *38*(3), 1–8.
Stern, D. N., Sander, L. W., Nahum, J. P., Harrison, A. M., Lyons-Ruth, K., Morgan, A. C., Bruschweiler-Stern, N., & Tronick, E. Z. (1998). Non-interpretive

mechanisms in psychoanalytic therapy. The "something more" than interpretation. The process of change study group. *The International Journal of Psycho-Analysis, 79*(Pt 5), 903–921.

Symington, N. (1993). *Narcissism: A new theory*. Karnac Books.

Symington, N. (2007). A technique for facilitating the creation of mind. *The International Journal of Psychoanalysis, 88*(6), 1409–1422. https://doi.org/10.1516/BN47-2657-886V-7256

Winnicott, D. W. (1971). *Playing and Reality. Routledge*. London and New York., 1991.

Winnicott, D. W. (2016). Mirror-role of mother and family in child development. In L. Caldwell & H. Taylor Robinson (Eds.), *The collected works of D. W. Winnicott: Volume 8, 1967–1968* (pp. 211–218). Oxford University Press. https://doi.org/10.1093/med:psych/9780190271404.003.0038

Wolf, E. S. (1994). Narcissistic lust and other vicissitudes of sexuality. *Psychoanalytic Inquiry, 14*(4), 519–534. https://doi.org/10.1080/07351699409534004

Chapter 6

Selfobject Needs as a Mirror of States of the Mind at Times of Environmental Threat and Discontent

Introduction

Following an analytic session, I received a message in which the patient wrote:

> *Thank you for the meeting today.*
>
> *I wish to share with you my experience of the meeting. . . . It felt as if sandpaper was rubbed on exposed skin. . . . It might appear smooth and even now, but it also feels chafed and raw. . . .*
>
> *We spoke about dissociation. Dissociation takes a high toll. We [she and I as therapists] know how to detect ruptures instantly, to fulfill our function and weave together that which is unraveled. The question that preoccupied me today was whether we can mend ruptures safely and to search delicately for the right approach so that we can reconnect disconnected positions in a curative way. . . .*
>
> *When you talked about my option to choose my (political) views, I felt that you were distancing yourself from me; you offered an alternative to my necessary dissociation too rapidly.*
>
> *How much time does it take before one can integrate dissociated parts? I know that the current events are difficult for you, too, but your perspective is different, and the gap between us may grow to be too wide. . . . Could we try to be together in this distress, bearing in mind the particular difficulties each of us faces?*

Times of discontent, such as wars, political upheaval, or the pandemic, expose analysts to unknown challenges. The external reality may arouse various responses both in the patients and in the analysts. Thus, the walls of the analytic setting are shaking and sometimes even falling. The analyst must

DOI: 10.4324/9781003449386-6

find ways to deal with a wide range of selfobject needs while being aware of her own mental fluctuations.

The chapter will focus on various clinical situations during the COVID-19 pandemic. These situations can represent clinical dilemmas at any time of environmental stress and discontent. The wars that occurred in Israel at different times presented very similar challenges for analysts. The key question is how to maintain the clinical setup when both analyst and patient are exposed to the same external threatening reality, and the analyst must manage the transferential manifestations that come up in this situation.

Three clinical vignettes describe different interactions in an unstable and unsafe analytic setting. It is remarkable how the patient's reactions to the stressful situation constitute the analyst's responses. The responses are entangled and lead at each time to a different dialogue.

The first vignette concerns a regressive state of the self. The patient cannot bear the analyst's vulnerability, her lack of immunity, and her inability to be totally centered around her needs. Archaic grandiosity and narcissistic rage are frequent manifestations in such situations. In this fragmented state, there is no faith in the analyst's ability to contain the situation properly. Therefore, the self must contain itself.

The second vignette relates to intensified twinship needs. Here, the patient mainly needs recognition and understanding of her existential situation, and the analyst tries to fulfill this selfobject function. The need to fulfill twinship functions was understood initially, in Kohut's thinking, as mirroring that cultivates grandiosity and was later defined as a separate selfobject transference.

The third situation illustrates the patient's lucid recognition of the current complexity. The patient maintains clarity of mind and is not too activated by environmental distress. The patient holds on to a transcendental position when her self is adequately supported by the analyst. In this case, it is possible to surrender to the tranquil analytic work.

Situation I: Archaic Grandiosity

A patient returned to the clinic after weeks of lockdown and a lack of face-to-face meetings. During lockdown we were continuously in touch by phone and seemed to maintain a consistent and intensive working relationship. Upon her return, she began by criticizing "people's unreasonable cautiousness." In her view, the pandemic posed no danger, and she thought that peoples' exaggerated cautiousness was an expression of fear, a "horror show," which they created in their imagination. "These cautious people are hypochondriacs," she added in a cynical tone. The conversation continued, and the patient ended the hour with a softly spoken comment: "No one protects me; I have to protect myself."

I pointed out the rage that had accumulated inside her due to our abrupt separation, as well as the sense of abandonment that she experienced. The lockdown had produced a sudden disruption of a delicate continuity of being and presence. The patient explained that the analysis should be above anything else and couldn't understand why I had agreed to exclude her during the lockdown. The clinic's wide open windows led her to wonder how I could possibly have "exposed" her to the unprotected public area. She was preoccupied with my betrayal of her, my preoccupation with my subjectivity, and not the pandemic.

The conversation quickly led to talk of early memories, images of her childhood, and the countless times when she felt that her parents urged her to engage in tasks that probably were a substitute for their own helplessness but, at the time, were beyond her. She described parents who ridiculed her moments of neediness by communicating that vulnerability was shameful and inappropriate. Step by step, the patient described how these humiliations led her to adopt omnipotent survival practices and apparent resilience to reinforce her own protective shell. From what the patient said, it was evident that her parents had not provided sufficient selfobject functions to enable her to cultivate an appropriate grandiosity, nor did they instill in her healthy narcissistic experiences, joy, and hope. What could have developed if she had seen a glimmer of admiration in her mother's eyes was crushed. Instead, due to her vulnerability and insecurity, she cultivated a kind of isolated arrogance, archaic omnipotence, and denial of the underlying emptiness that was in her mind.

Her excessive cynicism and rage left me speechless. I sensed the way in which the patient was dismissing my subjectivity. Kohut (1996) and Ana Ornstein (1998) relate to these situations of rage in analysis, when the patient's injured narcissism erases the subjectivity of the analyst and describes the possible complex consequences during such moments. This objectification of the analyst can evoke in him a type of rejection and even occasional aggression. His attentiveness is liable to be undermined, and his responses are likely to be artificial, flattened, a deceptive presentation that communicates that "everything is all right." Accumulated anger is liable to lead to a loss of patience and to a kind of rebuke. Kohut notes that only an analytic process that revitalizes the patient's healthy grandiosity is likely to moderate and alleviate the patient's negativity. Healthy grandiosity eliminates the defensive need to annul the other.

In the case under discussion here, I caved into a defensive approach and began to explain how keeping the room ventilated also protects the patient. I felt distanced from her, uncomfortable, perhaps even disgusted at her self-righteous approach, and I was sure that she would sense my feelings. Together, we were able to create a step-by-step reconstruction of the "needy" child and the "rejecting" parent. At the same time, given the awareness that it is a transferential attitude, I did my best to search for an understanding and a fitting intervention appropriate to her distress.

Patients do not easily give up childhood needs that were not fulfilled. They continue to demand what is due to them. I thought about Kohut's (1996) suggestion of relating to archaic grandiosity in an empathetic and positive way, in the same manner, that we relate to potential capacities that suddenly emerge and are at the disposal of the patient. In the main, it is important to help the patient to be aware and to cultivate his mental courage and efficacy, to give him the feeling that he has the possibility of influencing the analyst. Also, I remembered Winnicott's suggestion that the treatment of such patients requires extreme patience.

I told her that I would do everything I possibly could to ensure that the conditions in the clinic would suit her. Toward our next meeting, the sliding windows in the clinic, which had been removed, were back in their place. I tried to restore the confidence and inspiration felt in the room as an extension of a selfobject function.

This responsiveness may raise various questions: Was it the environmental distress that led the analyst to lose sight of her boundaries? Did the analyst act out of guilt for the hostility she felt toward the patient in her countertransference? Can the analyst's response be perceived as acting out and non-survival in the Winnicottian sense? Perhaps it would have been appropriate to suggest an interpretation that relates to what she said as an attack on the analytic relationship.

In the spirit of Kohut and Winnicott, we learn that those patients whose analysis demands coping with primitive emotional development require that the analyst properly examine his technique and understand that discontent stems from a repetition of primary environmental impingements. Understandably, for this patient, the interruption in the continuousness of the sessions and the widely open window were experienced as an empathic failure. Such cases require special patience and a particularly persistent environmental adaptation, which will enable the patient to nurture the core of her true self, as opposed to nurturing the shell, the false self. For the patient, the clinic is a mother's womb, a space that must be kept intact. We are reminded of what Winnicott (1992, p. 288, italics in the original) said:

> The couch and the pillows are there for the patient's use. They will appear in ideas and dreams and then will stand for the analyst's body. Breasts, arms, hands, etc, in an infinite variety of ways. In so far as the patient is regressed (for a moment, or for an hour or over a long period of time), the couch *is* the analyst; the pillows *are* breasts; the analyst is the mother at a certain past era.

This act of mine – returning the windows to their original place – was an entirely conscious and calculated act. In this context, the return of the windows is a non-verbal response, its significance being:

> I can see the cause of your suffering in the past as well as in the present. You feel that no one responded to your needs, However, now, despite the complex context in which we find ourselves, what you say is being heard. You can exert your influence on me.

This message incorporates a reference to past traumas alongside the communication that the present will be managed differently. The traumatic past is incorporated into the intervention, as well as the hope of a new beginning. The analyst is not attempting to regain control, nor does she interpret the patient's negativity. Instead, the analyst assumes responsibility for the patient's distress, probably in a Levinasian mode. This non-verbal intervention recognizes the patient's subjective experience of being deserted by those who should have functioned as selfobjects for her. By using a tone of speech lacking defensiveness or vindictiveness, she restores the patient's faith in selfobject functioning and her idealization of the analyst as an analytic mother who diverges from the archaic mother.

The intervention acknowledges the rigid and rudimental state of the self when fragmented. The patient's demandingness is understood as a revolt against past situations when she had to submit to others and disregard her own needs. Gratifying her needs at present validates, promotes, and constitutes them. The analyst accepts the patient as she is and refrains from "correcting" her. The important thing here is that need is rediscovered and recreated. The need system is reorganized.

Ghent (2001) distinguished between need and neediness. Need represents the interest of the healthy self, whereas neediness evolves from rejected needs. A regression to neediness is easily evoked within the transference relationship. In this context, Ghent (1990) also mentions the anatomy of Amea, as described by Doi (1973). Doi expands the thinking of Freud in regard to transference and refers to the Japanese psychology of dependence; the "passive" need of human beings to be cared for by those who are older, by teachers, by parents, as well as by analysts. Such care should consist of unspoken support; it does not require any interpretation, and it is appropriate to take it for granted. It is considered a universal human need. Surrender to a superior person realizes a fantasy of continuous selfobject functioning (Togashi, 2020). When this need is not met, demand evolves, gets more and more intense, and even becomes aggressive.

In our context, we can understand the demandingness of this patient in this context. In other words, it is important not to consider her attitude just as a manifestation of her aggressive drive but as an expression of a plea of a fragmented self that someone take responsibility for caring for her. More so, we can assume, in this case, that her insistence on support of her needs is a sight of emerging courage and assertiveness. Listening to her hidden plea and validating it nurtures the tentative seeds that may lead to the restoration of the self and the patient's area of faith.

Interestingly, the additional precautions I suggested taking during the pandemic's second wave were understood and accepted by the patient. The archaic grandiosity gave way to an understanding that we are all vulnerable, that our ability to control reality is limited, and that we are but two individuals in a line of others who accept the same safeguards. The analyst realized that her responsiveness during the first wave ultimately fostered an expansion of the patient's mind.

Situation II: Twinship

Transferences can assume a wide range of forms and transformations. The following vignette describes a situation in which patient and analyst may share a similar kind of psychic pain.

A patient tells me that her partner, who was supposed to come for the weekend from another town in which he lives, suddenly announced that he was unable to come because he had to help his elderly mother. The patient explains that relations with her partner are generally stable and that one could absolutely accept his decision as reasonable and understandable. However, on this occasion, it was not so. Her partner's message left her feeling pained, experiencing a terrible sense of abandonment, overwhelmed by inexplicable anger and disappointment, and at a loss to know how she would get through the weekend alone.

This patient is not in the grip of archaic grandiosity as was the previous patient, nor does she convert her distress into rage. She usually embraces painful situations and accepts them. In this case, the self is not trapped in a grandiose shell but rather lives and experiences the real suffering core. I knew that this disproportionate vulnerability saddened the patient a great deal. In general, she is excessively empathetic to the needs of others and regulates her own needs in a controlled, even restrained manner. Now, she is in an extremely disturbed state.

Her condition and the way she referred to her partner made it possible for us to be in the eye of the storm together. The patient explained that her response to the present situation was linked to previous relationships in which she always had to be "considerate" and the "responsible adult." She no longer wanted to play that role. Amid the disruptions and uncertainty of the COVID-19 period, whether at work or caring for her children, she was simply unable to put up with yet another unexpected change of plan. Her innate patience collapsed and turned into an unbearable sadness.

After years of analysis undertaken by this woman, it wasn't difficult to feel and even imagine her angst. In my mind, I saw an image of her at the beginning of her life. She had been placed in an orphanage because of her mother's weariness. The mother visited her, showered her, and in doing so, she detected bruises that no one had noticed before, treated them, and then left. The little girl didn't know when her mother would return. I went over this formative scene at the beginning of her life. We were able to see the disruptions caused by the mother alongside her being a mother who took care of her daughter with much devotion when she happened to be with her.

For a second, while we were both immersed in this reality of an abandoned toddler unable to know when or even whether her mother would return, a previous memory crept into my mind. When I was eight years old, my parents and I were in a foreign town. They had gone out in the evening and left me alone. I stood at the window for a seemingly endless hour waiting, clutching my doll Alisa with both hands. The memory flashed through my mind. I didn't know when they would return.

The patient was not expecting any kind of mirroring response nor an uplifting reaction. She just needed validation by an understanding other who would recognize her own subjectivity at that time. Without knowing what had gone through my mind, she spoke to a "twin" who need not respond. The most appropriate situation was for us to be together in silence, similar to the examples mentioned by Kohut: the girl who stands next to her grandmother in the kitchen, the boy who loves to "shave" next to his father in front of the mirror or work with his tools in the basement. In such situations, there is a profound, wordless, and uninterpreted understanding between two subjects.

It is important to note that in her transference, this patient is not experiencing the analyst as a disappointing object but rather as a participating subject. She does not project traumatic past experiences on the analytic situation (as is the case in classical transference) but rather encounters mutual regulation (Lachmann & Beebe, 1996) and co-creation of unknown experiences. The ability to feel pain in the presence of an other promotes the twinship transference, finding oneself in the other. The situation confirms to the patient that she is a human being among other human beings (Kohut, 1984). These situations exist not only in early childhood or regressive situations in later life but also in the context of normal day-to-day experiences. In these circumstances, memory traces can be rewritten and updated in line with the new shared experience.

Kohut believed that finding twinship relations is a natural human need. Usually, we assume that the patient is the one who searches for twinship between the analyst and herself. In our case, the analyst found a common link between herself and the patient in her mind and surrendered to this empathic experience. We may wonder: Do we need to find similarities between us and our patients to constitute empathy? Self psychology usually maintains that such similarities are not needed since we are not looking for identity or for identification. Still, it is reasonable to believe that constituting some resemblance in the mind of the analyst supports the constitution of an empathic stance.

Twinship as a basic human need is not recognized in mainstream psychoanalytic literature. Referencing twinship transferences expands psychoanalytic thinking and diverts it from its main interest, personal traumas, to a broad perspective that relates to a universal conception in regard to human vulnerability. Cherished moments in analysis are instances when we dare to touch an absolute reality that goes beyond the individual, consists of an area of faith, and, at the same time, captures the uncertainties of life. Such moments open the mind to the complexities of our reality and promote the renunciation of dichotomies.

Neville Symington, in his book *The Making of a Psychotherapist* (1996), devotes a chapter to the subject of psychic pain and moral courage. He suggests that there is a universal truth according to which all animals, including humans, try to avoid mental and physical pain. Symington suggests that those who try to avoid dealing with emotional pain are doomed to remain immature and emotionally undeveloped. He claims that coping with psychic pain requires courage and is facilitated by the presence of an understanding other: "*Real pain is always connected to self-knowledge that comes through another*" (Symington, 1996, p. 60, italics added). Relieving the patient from her psychic pain requires the analyst to have the courage to sketch, as clearly as possible, a picture explaining the source of the pain, staying with her patient as she faces up to the ensuing emotional storm. The personal memory that crept into my mind in the course of that hour, outside awareness, is an image that elucidated the subjective experience of the patient and enabled her to feel understood.

Situation III: Lucidity, Compassion, and Transcendence

In this third situation, clarity of mind is maintained despite the disturbing external reality. Surrender alleviated suffering and enabled a focus on a creative inner reality.

The second wave of the COVID-19 pandemic led me to suggest that my patients and I should wear masks inside the consulting room. Naturally, the suggestion concerned me; I thought it might bring to the surface once more the alienation that was experienced during the first wave and, in that sense, could lead to a kind of re-traumatization. At the same time, I felt that to be calm and focused and not go back to Zoom or the phone, this was the appropriate move. I expected my suggestion to arouse difficulty and resistance, but to my surprise, within a few minutes of dealing with the discomfort involved in wearing the mask, we got used to the situation, and during most clinical hours, we were able to truly engage in the analytic work without reference to the environmental difficulties that surrounded us.

One morning, a patient entered my room, and I suddenly found myself delaying wearing my mask, looking at her for what seemed like a long time, enabling her to look at me and see my face. We inspected each other for a few long moments. We then put on our masks. During this particular moment, I clearly felt that wearing the mask recreates a sort of alienation, a barrier, a disowning of unmediated "togetherness," and shared this feeling with her in a friendly and even somewhat joking tone, as if to say: "What a bummer." Conceivably, this intervention was intended to enable a referral to a possible sense of estrangement, which may have remained unspoken but nonetheless felt by both of us. I was surprised to hear the patient's response: "Let's leave that alone; what somebody's face looks like is not important." She lay on the couch and began telling me about a dream she had.

Clearly, one could think that the patient, as a parental child or as one who was disavowing reality, was trying to calm me down. My impression, however, was that she was communicating something like: "Stop worrying about that; it is a side issue." I understood that the patient was already immersed in her inner reality, whereas I was still preoccupied with issues that were related to the external reality. Conceivably, she was able to preserve a lucid mind that does not argue with the situation, is not particularly attached to the difficulties involved, and is not drawn to them. Such lucidity is possible where the analytic relation is well-founded and undisputed.

This patient was blessed with remarkable equanimity, a state of mental balance and mindfulness in which it is possible to face different situations openly, without defensiveness, including adversaries or anxiety. Therefore, the patient did not feel the need to discuss the matter of the mask and analyze it any further. In her wisdom, she accepted that there was a certain situation at this moment and understood that there would be different situations at other moments. She accepted the principle of transience and did not dispute it. Her expanded mind enabled her to focus on her inner world without external interference.

The concept of transience is mentioned by various psychoanalysts. In 1916, Freud wrote his paper "On Transience" and referred to the loss of the beauty of nature when the winter would come and the proneness of decay of all that is beautiful and perfect. He vehemently disputed this pessimistic idea and suggested that scarcity raises the value of the moment: "As regards the beauty of nature, each time it is destroyed by winter it comes back again next year, so that in relation to the length of our lives it can in fact be regarded as eternal" (Freud, 1957, p. 305). The subtext was his evolving interest in morning and melancholia. Freud suggested that the ability to mourn is a significant achievement of the ego. It is linked to the capacity to accept losses, not remain melancholically attached to them, owing to an ability of renunciation.

Already in his earlier 1912 article "Recommendations to Physicians Practicing Psychoanalysis," Freud (1958) suggested that doctors not exert themselves attempting to remember certain things. Rather, they should simply listen with even free-floating attention. Doctors should not be fixated on particular situations. Fixations simply limit the scope of analytic freedom.

Bion (1988), in his paper "Notes on Memory and Desire," takes this statement of Freud's further and gives it an added meaning. Without any direct reference to Freud's work, he actually repeats the principle of even free-floating attention, which seeks to include everything that comes to mind at a certain moment. Like Freud, he warns against clinging to what is known in advance and suggests that meaning emerges in the absence of a preconceived form. Bion (1984) goes further and describes the apparently paradoxical idea of "thoughts without a thinker" as follows: "Thoughts exist without a thinker. The idea of infinitude is prior to any idea of finite. The finite is won from the dark and formless infinite" (p. 165). This idea encompasses an assumption that there is an infinity of floating thoughts that have not yet been considered.

This is a quantum idea in the sense that it does not mark any fixed beginning or a definite ending to phenomena. Every phenomenon or thought is found in an infinite sequence of what existed before it and what will come after it. Man, like a butterfly hunter, catches this or that thought at a certain moment, depending on the lucidity of his mind. This conception also consists in the idea of "the Grid" (Bion, 1989), which signifies a constant change of thoughts, from beta to alpha and from alpha toward clear abstract thinking, and alternatively, the "retreat" of thought to its obscure places. Thoughts and experiences are in constant flux between clarity and obscurity.

While Freud described impermanence as the nature of things that must be accepted without clinging to what is lost, and Bion referred to the endless changeability of thoughts, Kohut proposed the idea of transience as one possible way to transform archaic narcissism into mature narcissism. Accepting impermanence implies the infinite potential inherent in the self, and the different dispositions that the self can assume in different contexts. Thus, changes are no longer seen as loss or as bringing disaster to the self, but rather they are seen as a phenomenon of infinite entanglement between different situations. The third example illustrates this state of mind.

Concluding Remarks

Three examples illustrate different selfobject needs that arise under conditions of environmental threat. The first example describes a regressive reaction, which is characterized by archaic grandiosity and narcissistic rage, as a way to deal with feelings of lack of perspective, depression, and hopelessness. The transferential matrix is shaken, and the idealization of the analyst is undermined when a patient cannot tolerate the fact that she is not immune to the threats of reality. The patient's distress is met with an accepting response that reconstitutes the analyst's position as an idealized selfobject.

The second example describes a situation where the patient needs more than anything understanding and recognition of her current situation. From the dawn of her childhood, she exists in a world of unsettling insecurity. The analyst embraces this need through her attentive presence and promotes an experience of twinship in her mind. This transformation, in the analyst's mind, elevates the patient's suffering and restores the fragmented self.

The third example describes a patient whose mind is clear enough that she is not activated by the invasive trauma. This occurs when the selfobject functions are well constituted, and the analyst's constant presence is internalized. In this case, compassion emerges and enables the patient to accept the situation and not be drawn to the distress caused by the external reality. The analytic work is carried out mindfully.

Psychoanalysis can no longer be content with discussing the inner world and classical transference alone. A traumatic reality that penetrates the consulting room can consume at once the things taken for granted in our lives and negate the assumption that the world is safe and known. Traumatic realities may connect us to our humane vulnerability, to the limitations and transience of life. These threatening situations trigger different selfobject needs, depending on the degree of narcissistic development of the patients. Those whose narcissism is archaic react very differently from those whose narcissism is mature and whose mind is lucid. These different selfobject needs challenge the analyst and his ability to weave a unique space and a new beginning for each and every patient.

References

Bion, W. (1984). *Second thoughts: Selected papers on psycho-analysis*. Karnac Books.

Bion, W. R. (1988). Notes on memory and desire. In E. B. Spillius (Ed.), *Melanie Klein today: Developments in theory and practice: Vol. 2: Mainly practice* (pp. 17–21). Routledge.

Bion, W. R. (1989). *Two papers: The grid and caesura*. Karnac Books.

Doi, T. (1973). *The anatomy of dependence* (Revised ed.). Kodansha International.

Freud, S. (1957). On transience. In J. Stachley & A. Freud (Eds.), *The standard edition of the complete psychological works of Sigmund Freud: Vol. 14 (1914–1916): On the history of the psycho-analytic movement, papers on metapsychology and other works* (pp. 303–307). Hogarth Press.

Freud, S. (1958). Recommendations to physicians practicing psycho-analysis. In J. Strachley & A. Freud (Eds.), *The standard edition of the complete psychological works of Sigmund Freud: Vol. 12 (1911–1913): The case of schreber papers on technique & other works* (pp. 109–120). Hogarth Press.

Ghent, E. (1990). Masochism, submission, surrender: Masochism as a perversion of surrender. *Contemporary Psychoanalysis*, *26*(1), 108–136. https://doi.org/10.1080/00107530.1990.10746643

Ghent, E. (2001). Need, paradox, and surrender: Commentary on paper by Adam Phillips. *Psychoanalytic Dialogues*, *11*(1), 23–41. https://doi.org/10.1080/10481881109348595

Kohut, H. (1984). *How does analysis cure?* (A. Goldberg & P. Stepansky, Eds.). University of Chicago Press.

Kohut, H. (1996). *Heinz Kohut: The Chicago institute lectures* (P. Tolpin & M. Tolpin, Eds.). Routledge.

Lachmann, F. M., & Beebe, B. (1996). The contribution of self- and mutual regulation to therapeutic action: A case illustration. In A. I. Goldberg (Ed.), *Progress in self psychology. Vol. 12: Basic ideas reconsidered* (pp. 123–140). Routledge.

Ornstein, A. (1998). The fate of narcissistic rage in psychotherapy. *Psychoanalytic Inquiry*, *18*(1), 55–70. https://doi.org/10.1080/07351699809534170

Symington, N. (1996). *The making of a psychotherapist*. Karnac Books.

Togashi, K. (2020). *The psychoanalytic zero: A decolonizing study of therapeutic dialogues*. Routledge.

Winnicott, D. W. (1992). *Through paediatrics to psycho-analysis: Collected papers*. Karnac Books.

Chapter 7

Accepting Transience

Relinquishment of the Ego or an Expansion of the Mind?*

Introduction

It is assumed that the preoccupation with the principle of transience is linked to maturity in the latter years of life. When the prospect of impending death is experienced, we experience losses, disappointments, and traumas, as well as diminishing pleasures. "We have lived," and at a certain moment in time, we have to part from parents, from children, from friends, from work, and from physical functioning because of the possibility of our own death hovering or because of the circumstances in which those final years of life are spent. At a certain moment, the era of innocence ends. Confidence and complacency make way for doubts and uncertainty. And the realization that nothing is permanent; there is a sense that at any moment, everything may succumb to transience and no longer be.

Freud (1957b) wrote his paper "On Transience" in the middle of World War I. At the time, he was also losing the support of his faithful student Carl Jung, who abandoned the thinking of his mentor in favor of his own version of transience. In "On Transience," Freud describes either a real or imaginary summer walk with Lou Andreas-Salomé and Rainer Maria Rilke, then a young poet. Salomé and Rilke were complaining about nature's beauty, which would end with the onset of autumn. Freud observed nature's short-lived beauty and suggested that clinging to it and the preoccupation with its loss were disturbing the enjoyment and excitement of the splendor of the moment. He suggests that one's observation should reflect a faith that the world will be rebuilt after the war, perhaps in a better way.

Freud offers two possible ways of responding to transience. One is the diminution of the value of the lost object, a certain non-attachment out of

* An earlier version of this chapter in Hebrew was published as Mann (2017).

DOI: 10.4324/9781003449386-7

the fear of its loss. Alternatively, Freud suggests a denial of the passage of time, a sort of illusion that he links to desire. These two possible responses, lessening the value of the object or denial of the passage of time, are a means of avoiding pain. These two forms of defensive mechanisms protect against the need to mourn. Freud claims that the ability to mourn is a significant achievement of the ego, that it is connected to the ability to relinquish, to bear losses in the course of non-melancholic reasonable mourning, resembling Klein's later thinking on the depressive position.

A year later, in 1917, Freud (1957a) wrote "Mourning and Melancholia" yet another discussion about loss and the various ways of processing it. In this paper, Freud writes about healthy mourning, a period during which we internalize aspects of the lost object and turn them into permanent representations of the object in the ego. He distinguishes between healthy mourning and melancholia, a state of mind in which we are unable to internalize the object but remain attached to and cling to it. In such a case, the ego drowns in the shadow of the object and is unable to transform the lost object into a mental representation, develop, and release the external object. The ego cannot give up and accept transience and so remains immersed in the lost object.

One can undoubtedly see a continuum between these Freudian ideas.

Does the value of the object change because of transience? The interesting and paradoxical claim by Freud in his paper is that transience does not alter the value of the lost object and certainly does not lessen its worth. The reverse is the case. Transient objects in fact are possibly more valuable precisely because of their transience. Thus, Freud reinforced the importance of transience, its special value to be found here, now, at this moment, in the present.

In his book *Transforming Narcissism* (2007), Frank Lachmann discussed "disorders of temporality" manifested by fear of death, alienation, distancing from reality, momentary experiences, and fixation on certain situations. All of these are viewed by Lachmann as ways of denying transience by means of dissociative mechanisms and the flattening of the subjective experience of pain due to loss. In other words, they are ways of clinging to certain situations and an unwillingness to accept necessary changes. This attachment can be thought of as a grandiosity that cannot be relinquished. That is, desperately holding on to life or what a person has in his life is a manifestation of narcissistic grandiosity. Consequently, loss turns into a crushing blow to grandiosity. We can see fears of death as well as a refusal to make other concessions, as belonging to the axis of grandiosity, the fear of losing control over what there is.

On the other hand, there is a line of thought that regards a profound acceptance of transience as an ideal. Here, transience is not perceived as loss nor as the cause of a disaster imposed on the self. Instead, it is thought that even if the particular individual self ceases to exist or changes, the ideal will continue to exist, though in a different manner. Such a position recognizes the acceptance of transience without trauma and without the collapse of the self. This line of thought leads us to Heinz Kohut's reflections.

In his important canonical paper, "Forms and Transformation of Narcissism" (1966), Kohut courageously suggests the transformation of archaic narcissism to a mature form of narcissism, which he describes as supra-individual narcissism or cosmic narcissism. In other words, archaic narcissism is transformed into a configuration that goes beyond the personal interest of the individual. Kohut referred to five possible forms of transformations to cosmic narcissism: "creativity, empathy, acceptance of impermanence, humor, and wisdom" (Kohut, 1966).

Lachmann (2007) invites us to use Kohut's seminal paper as an updated springboard to the investigation of narcissism's fluctuations and its possible transformations. At the same time, Lachmann claims that Kohut did not indicate the way in which these transformations can be realized and what is required to make them happen. He suggests that we refer to this ambiguous part of Kohut's teachings and claims that a treatment that strives to achieve such transformations should consist of them as part of the process itself. Which is to say that if the therapist–patient relationship is based on these five principles, it can be assumed that they will be internalized elements in the process of psychic change that the patient undergoes, functions that he will acquire for himself during the healing process.

However, while to some extent it is possible to demonstrate the nature of creativity, empathy, humor, and wisdom and to see that these functions are indeed acquired in therapy, it seems rather difficult to demonstrate the principle of the acceptance of transience. Indeed, a review of the various materials we have studied over the years revealed that there was relatively limited discussion of this principle. Whenever this dimension was referred to, it was only in the context of what Kohut had originally referred to, namely the acceptance of the transience of life. It is interesting to note that Kohut himself, in the summary of his article on the transformations of narcissism and the changes in personality that occur as a result of the treatment, lists all four other transformations and omits the transformation triggered by accepting transience. One wonders why he did not mention it. Could it be that it was too metaphysical for him? Was it perhaps too frightening or too complex as a transformation for it to be realized in therapy? For now, we have no alternative other than to leave these questions open to further discussion.

What I have written here thus far is directed at Kohut's studies of the issue of transience, as developed in the course of various stages in his thinking. Later, I will offer a broadening of this view of transience that will also include the transience of the states of the self, albeit without them being anchored in the context of the transience of life. One can think about the transience of the self-states, of the self's internalizations, of the transience between the appearance of the soma and the psyche, and, finally, being a transient/changing selfobject with various patients and in different circumstances. All these are variant modes of being within the potentiality of the same self in its various contexts.

Kohut – On Transience

Transience of self-states is a theoretical idea anchored in the heart of self psychology. Kohut related to the movement between formation and potential, between the virtual formation and the cohesive form. The virtual can assume innumerable possible forms into which it can collapse; each one is liable to be temporary and transient. Each of these forms is constituted by a particular state of narcissistic development.

We can assume that fluctuations of these forms and transformations can be explained by quantum theory. A quantum state indicates that the self-state infinitely changes among countless emergings which occur at various times, inspired by contextual circumstances. The vast potentiality is the reservoir of all the possible variations. Thus, the concept of transience is anchored in the assumption that all the appearances belong to the same cosmos. This infinite cosmos can be apprehended only rarely and just momentarily in extraordinary moments of lucidity. Most of the time, we see only its appearances, waves, particles, and then again waves. Such a view is contrary to theories that believe in multiple selves, asserting that these selves exist simultaneously, each one with its own subjectivity and an intersubjectivity between them. The understanding in self psychology is that we seek to identify the various subjective realities of the same elemental self. It is interesting that even Philip Bromberg (2006), who described various self-identities, suggests that self-unity captures the experience of our being fully in life.[1]

It seems to me that the first signs of interest in the question of transience are already to be found in Kohut's (1984) discussion of transmuting internalization. Kohut was preoccupied by the question of how the presence of an other can arouse the emergence of "new" functions in the self. He discusses the internalization that takes place when the connection to the selfobject activates new functions within the self. This transformation of the self occurs in the presence of a mirroring and ideal selfobject. The selfobject's function undergoes a process of transmuting internalization and becomes a new permanent structural quality within the self. Kohut, being still faithful to his psychoanalytic heritage, is captivated by the model of psychic structures.

In his 1966 paper, Kohut, previously a believer in ego psychology, suggests that the self is not merely a representation within the ego but maintains that the self is an entity far larger than the structure, the ego (perhaps similarly to Jung's perception of the self). The refined self can be coherent and mature and, furthermore, can be integrated and cosmic. In this instance, the self relinquishes its permanent dimensions and dissolves into an impermanent cosmic selfhood that does not have its place in something permanent and definable but is, in and of itself, empty of content (Kulka, 2005). Thus, Kohut offers a quantum leap beyond cohesion and beyond the intrapsychic structures that characterize the teachings of Freud and the neo-Freudians. We may describe this new dimension as a "trans-psychic" state. The self, in its extensions, is profoundly linked to the universe, to the world, and all that it comprises. This transcendence annuls the ontological

1 In *Awakening the Dreamer*, Bromberg (2006) writes:

> Regardless of the extent of dissociation, when the therapist is able to relate to each aspect of the patient's self in terms of its own subjectivity, each part becomes increasingly able to coexist with the rest and in that sense is more subjectively linked to others. This linking of self-states necessarily increases a person's sense of wholeness, but the active ingredient in treatment that makes this possible is human relatedness. Self-unity, the mysterious force that holds selfhood together and permits the coexistence of self-continuity and self-coherence across self-states is made possible by what happens between people. Ultimately, self-unity is a shorthand term for the experience of being fully in life – life being our connection with the rest of humanity. And in therapy the patient's connectedness with humanity is lived by being fully in the relational experience with the therapist, and vice.
>
> (p. 27)

identity and creates a mirror consciousness which neither refuses nor does it cling to anything. It reflects what *is* at that very moment and changes accordingly. Kohut (1966) notes specifically that in certain psychological states, the boundaries of the self may expand far beyond the borders of the individual, or it may shrink and become reduced to a single one of its goals.

Kohut suggests that both the horizontal and the vertical split become apparent when the self is fragmented, reduced. Split self-states are not the primordial natural situations of a baby in a state of total immersion with his mother. Transformation to transience requires transcendence, abandoning the ruptures, and relinquishing attachments so as to enable the extension of the self beyond its boundaries, similar to the pre-traumatic baby. Here, the self ceases to exist as a particular entity but can be an all-embracing selfhood:

> There exist, however, a number of acquisitions of the ego which, although genetically and dynamically related to the narcissistic drives . . . and which . . . must be evaluated not only as transformations of narcissism but even more as attainments of the ego and as attitudes and achievements of the personality.
>
> (Kohut, 1966, p. 257)

Kohut lists the five transformations, which include a person's ability to reflect on his own transience: "Man's capacity to acknowledge the finiteness of his existence, and to act in accordance with this painful discovery, may well be his greatest psychological achievement" (Kohut, 1966, p. 264). He suggests that the acceptance of transience is attained by the ego, which facilitates separation. Without this effort, one cannot reach a valid conceptualization of time, of boundaries, and of the inconstancy of object-attachments. He proposes that it is more difficult to emotionally acknowledge our own impermanence than to accept the object's inconsistency of existence.

> I have little doubt that those who are able to achieve this ultimate attitude towards life do so on the strength of a new, expanded, transformed narcissism: a cosmic narcissism which has transcended the bounds of the individual. . . . In any event, the genuine shift of the cathexes toward a cosmic narcissism is the enduring creative result of the steadfast activities of an autonomous ego, and only a very few are able to attain it.
>
> (Kohut, 1966, p. 266)

Here, Kohut distinguishes transience between individual narcissism and narcissism that transcends the individual, which he terms cosmic narcissism. The idea is borrowed from quantum physics – a theory that Kohut regarded as a fountainhead of inspiration. This conception resonates with the notion in physics about wave–particle duality. Differing appearances and a profound entanglement between them. We are reminded of Winnicott's wondering as to why we see separateness in the world where it does not exist.

A few months before his death, in his article "Introspection, Empathy, and the Semi-Circle of Mental Health" (1981), Kohut elaborated on the meaning of transience. The paper discusses the possibility of an unstructured, timeless existence in which one generation can share the joy of the next generation and let the next generation be a natural, nonconflictual continuation of the previous one. This kind of deep unity between generations is the nature of things.[2] Only where a split in that natural order occurs and pathology of the self dominates, as demonstrated by the myth of Oedipus, do intergenerational conflict and resentment emerge.

Kohut contrasts the myth of Oedipus with that of Odysseus. This later myth allows for a different perspective, namely viewing the next generation as an extension of the existing generation's self. Here, the particular narcissism of the young generation is seen as an expansion of the previous generation. Yet there is "a slip of the pen" in this suggestion: claiming that the next generation will resemble its predecessor implies that it will not be completely free to become itself. Do we detect in this remark a concealed collapse of the supra-individual approach? Is the next generation in fact a Freudian baby that has to serve the interest of the parental generation, or is it truly free to be an Odyssean baby that focuses on its own needs and that alone? In any event, Kohut praises generational transience. He openly and unequivocally believes that the supreme objective, and one which is extremely difficult to achieve, is participation in a world in which transience is recognized.

Kohut, in an interview with the theologian Robert L. Randall, which took place in March–April 1981, six months before his death (Strozier, 2001), offered his thoughts about death more distinctly, advancing a clear step further in his thinking about death and transience in general. At this point in time, his thoughts were not limited to the subject of death but linked

2 See an expanded discussion of this matter in Chapter 11.

transience to a broad world order. We can see Kohut moving from his observations on transience as a painful discovery to viewing transience as a source of joy and a mental achievement:

> There is a seed, there is a flowering, there is a wilting, there is death, and the next generation of roses takes over. I think that one isn't really fully alive if one doesn't somehow, down deep in one's bones, feel this eternal rhythm of life, this coming and going of which one is only a link in a chain. To me, this is an uplifting thought, not a discouraging thought. It goes beyond my individuality to something broader and more enduring than this little me that is common, hasn't been here during Plato's time, and will not be here in a thousand years when there's another Plato or maybe nothing. Who knows? Why do I have to be and have been around? I wasn't, and I won't. That doesn't discourage me.
>
> (Strozier, 2001, p. 331)

We see that toward the end of his life, Kohut realized that besides the importance of cohesiveness and the formation of the self, the meaning of life goes beyond cohesiveness. This meaning links our particular lives to an endless chain of interconnected events and occurrences. Reverberations of this perspective can be found in the paper "On Courage" (written in the early 1970s). Kohut's position not only emphasizes death but also includes his latter-day thoughts on infinity. This dimension in Kohut's writing was not central to his thinking most of the time and was abandoned after his 1966 paper. This dimension has certainly not been accorded appropriate recognition. Moreover, it was omitted and neglected in the neo-Kohutian literature until scholars such as Max Sucharov (1992, 2001), Kulka (2005, 2010), Orange (2006), Mann (2013), and Togashi (2020) returned it to center stage. It can be assumed that the ideas of Robert Stolorow et al. (1987) and the system theories of Joe Lichtenberg et al. (2011) also strived for a broader perception and pointed to an infinite variability which transcends the individual in different ways.

It may well be that Kohut himself was insecure and slightly embarrassed by these unique positions of his; he may have sensed their "strangeness" and the uneasiness they might arouse among his professional colleagues. Even so, the discussion of transience is the most courageous of his contributions, and it is appropriate that it be accorded the place it deserves. Winnicott's (1953) thoughts on the transitional phenomenon validate these ideas and open a new psychoanalytic perspective to dealing with these metaphysical issues.

Thich Nhat Hanh (2001), a Vietnamese monk and an important Buddhist teacher who lived in France, showed his audience a cup of tea and asked what was in the cup. The immediate answer was, of course, "tea." And where did the tea come from? – from the thermos. And where did the thermos water come from? – from the river. Thus, when one looks at the tea, one sees the thermos, the river, the rain, and the clouds that brought the rain. Similarly, when people die, they do not disappear from the world but change the form of their presence. In the words of Yolanda Gampel (2010), they remain within us: "The parents who live through me." Things do not begin to be nor cease to be but appear under certain circumstances and cease to be present when the conditions change. Thus, even when things are not visible to the eye, they still exist as a seed within the reservoir of our consciousness, which can be watered or dried. Hence, the questions of where I came from and where I am going are deceptive questions. In reality, there is no place you came from, nor is there a place you will go to. There is only a current transient formation within a huge integrated field. The exercise is to give the rejected thoughts a place similar to that of the accepted thoughts to allot all thoughts the same potential.

We instigate every moment of the present through the way we perceive it: we do not create an entity from nothing, but we influence the existing by embracing or suspending it. This is how we impact the flow of things. Every present moment is an opportunity to validate what exists and enrich the experience with new content as a new beginning. Alternatively, it is an opportunity to suspend the existing and detach ourselves from it. It seems to me that this is the most profound way of applying the concept of transience.

Transience: Infinity of the Self with Reference to Bion

Bion's (1989) idea of "the Grid," a network that describes the flow of thoughts within the therapeutic hour, is defined as a constantly changing process. From beta elements that are unthinkable, there is an evolution to alpha elements: dreams, myths, and preconceptions, which lead to conceptions, further on to a concept, and finally to an algebraic calculus – the ultimate abstraction of thought.

However, as soon as the conception/concept is formulated, the emotional constellation will have already changed, returning us to a previous state of thinking. There will always be the to-and-fro between clarity of the mind and obfuscations. Thoughts are always changeable. It is therefore important not to cling to any particular position. Even so, every new thought is ostensibly derived in a profound way from an ancient intuitive understanding, in myths, in endless precedents that are mostly forgotten and yet are transmitted as a legacy in the passage of time from generation to generation. An invisible invariant, which Bion denotes as O. A well-known example of Bion's O is linked to the practice of painting. One can paint a field of sunflowers in different ways: realistically as flowers, as smooth yellow surfaces (resembling Mark Rothko's paintings), as bright spots of color as would an impressionist, as squares in the cubist style, or as endless other possible variations. Whatever the painting turns out to be, the various versions all consist of an invariant, which derives from an inner intuitive comprehension of the essence of things. This invariant is a latent content that is constituted by countless unknown sources, which do not necessarily coincide with the visible manifestation.

At the end of his days, Bion went further in his thinking. In his last paper, "Making the Best of a Bad Job," written in 1977, he wrote:

> I dislike terms that imply "the body" and "the mind," therefore I use the "Self" to include what I call body or mind, and "a mental space" for further ideas which may be developed. The philosophical statement of the approach is Monism.
>
> (Bion, 1977, p. 250)

Bion's contemplative writings offer a whole set of examples of these phenomena, situations in which apparent different occurrences stem from the same deep unity. For example, in his last paper, he writes about the prenatal as opposed to the postnatal parts of the personality. If Kohut wrote about the different self-states (virtual self, nuclear self, cohesive self, cosmic self) or the link between chains of generations, similarly, Bion described the quantum chain of the various personality modalities, including the link between the prenatal embryonic life and life after birth. He draws our attention to Freud's observation in *Inhibitions, Symptoms and Anxiety* (written in 1926): "There is much more continuity between intra-uterine life and earliest infancy than the impressive caesura of the act of birth would have us believe." Bion explains that Freud's summary can be understood as one in which the "impressive caesura" is too impressive to allow us to suppose that the fetus might have a proto-mind and personality or could develop its proto-mind into a mind after birth.

However, Bion (1989) is convinced that despite the apparent split between the prenatal part of the personality and the personality of the newborn, there is a significant continuity and affinity between the prenatal and postnatal minds. The first is endowed with archaic origins and is equipped with unique primordial intuitions, ones that can sense emotional fluctuations within the amniotic fluid and are not capable of thinking.[3] He suggests that in analysis, we see a total personality that has at some time, consciously or unconsciously, chosen a particular vertex from which to see the view. This total personality includes everything – prenatal aspects, newborn aspects, as well as mature aspects of the personality.

The model of prenatal and postnatal parts replaced the previous model of psychotic and nonpsychotic parts of the personality. In his last book, *A Memoir of the Future* (1991), Bion emphasized the significance of the prenatal parts and described them as not in any way psychotic. In fact, he views them as being endowed with talent and creativity: for instance, we find the intuitor of danger, the opponent of birth, one who prefers to have no interest in the external world and is at odds with those who deny the prenatal parts. There is a linguistic struggle between the parts, similar to the confusion of tongues in the myth of the Tower of Babel. It is interesting and relevant that Bion exalts these prenatal parts and suggests that we could regard artists, musicians, scientists, and discoverers as those who have dared to entertain these transitive thoughts and ideas. It is in the course of transit, in the course of changing from one position to another, that these people seem to be most perceptive and capable of tolerating a wide range of human behaviors that others disavow and reject.

Bion points to the prenatal parts, those experienced through the body, as opposed to the developed parts, those experienced through the mind – as belonging to the same self. Bion's successors, such as Elizabeth Bianchedi et al. (2002), elaborate on this perspective and suggest that we should not neglect those parts that have "fetal intuition." We must think about using those parts in the service of a mature and thinking self. More importantly,

3 Amniotic fluid is a primordial environment that does not belong to the mind. This is where physical-intuitive senses develop, for example the sense of smell, which later can develop into a function of thinking. The idea is that the body and the mind create language. Although these languages are sometimes seen as a developmental continuum, they can also be seen as complementing each other. Sometimes the body will speak, when the mind is prevented from expressing itself, when thoughts lack a thinker, and sometimes the mind will speak, if it becomes possible for matters to become thoughts.

we should not deprive ourselves of the rich and creative language of those primitive parts; they must be given precedence over the transience of the mature parts so that we don't miss out on their inspiring language. Attention to the less familiar parts of the self, those that have not yet been "socialized," actually opens a window of opportunity to novel and refreshing ideas. Omitting them or reducing their value depletes the wealth of the self.[4]

It transpired that the self does not consist of a fixed and stable entity. In differing circumstances, it takes on different manifestations: sometimes, it distorts itself, puts on a defensive armor, or communicates via the body. In another context, the self may change its appearance from fragile to cohesive, from false to real or vice versa. In all instances, it is still the same elemental self. This can be demonstrated simply by the chameleon, which changes its colors in different environments but never ceases to be a chameleon, even when its appearance changes. In fact, the changeability of its colors is its unique being. Another example, also quite a simple one, is the example of the islands in the sea. Islands appear to be different entities and separate from each other. If we removed the seawater, we would discover instead one continuous stretch surface area, albeit at different elevations.

I hope that these examples illustrate to some extent the radical idea of transience as part of a broad unity. A feeling of separateness exists at a certain moment by merely seeing it as a distinct phenomenon. This is the appearance of a particular particle, and it is important and significant. However, the discrete particle that emerges at one moment in time and in a certain context may transform and connect to a wider existence, to which it belongs in a profound existential sense.

Rosanna's Case: The Oak Tree and the Reeds

> The oak tree boasted to the reeds that it was stronger and more powerful than them, but then a windstorm approached, uprooting the big tree, while the reeds moved in tandem with the wind, bent with it, and remained embedded without being damaged. Does this mean that the reeds relinquished their egos, or were they endowed with a broader mindfulness?

Rosanna was in treatment for about seven years. At work, she dealt with juvenile delinquency. She came into therapy when her son, who was about

4 Similarly, Kohut (1985), in his conversations with Charles Strozier, mentions anthropology, which does appreciate the treatment of ancient cultures as primitive or less successful.

to enlist in the army, was emotionally unstable. Among other things, he complained to the police about her husband's alleged violence toward him. The father was not physically violent. He was abusive, humiliating his son in the presence of friends. Rosanna, watching from the sidelines, was a silent witness. Our work around these matters was complicated and often led us to rocky roads. Over time, we realized that in fact both her husband and Rosanna had abusive parents, a fact that Rosanna did not in any way associate with her son's situation. Rosanna was surprised and even amazed by this failure of recognition. This event became a metaphor between the two of us, an indicator of her inability at times to empathize with her children despite her conscious efforts to be a different parent than her parents.

This condition illustrates a vertical split, which is based on a narcissistic structure, where certain experiences are amplified and experienced as absolute truth, while other experiences, those that produce narcissistic vulnerability, are disavowed and rejected. The rejected experiences permeate the protection of the horizontal split. The process of restoring the split self will occur through the narcissistic nurturing of the damaged self, so that the rejection will no longer be a necessary defense mechanism and will facilitate the emergence into awareness of disavowed contents. We endured painful moments before we were able to regain clarity of mind.

After two more years in therapy, the subject of Rosanna's son becoming religious and turning to extremist circles became a concern. He moved his residence close to his Rabbi, who was involved in every aspect of his life. The son decided to immerse himself in religious studies during the day and a vocational course in the evening. This was immediately understood by the patient and her husband as an intermediate step toward an orthodox lifestyle of learning instead of working.

This decision was not in line with the family's way of life, its values, or its patterns of behavior. Rosanna's husband is secular with a love of life and recoils from any form of religious coercion. He was shocked and horrified by his son's decisions, while Rosanna, acting as a mediator between them, avoided confrontation in an attempt to maintain relative domestic peace.

Rosanna described the trip with her son on the eve of the Jewish New Year to Bnei Brak (a town largely populated by very orthodox Jews) to help him move his belongings to a community house for men who had decided to become religious. On their way, they traveled through the city center. Her son mentioned that he should call the guy with whom he would be sharing a room so that he could vacate the room before their arrival. Rosanna wondered why such a warning was necessary. Her son explained that extremely orthodox Jews were prohibited from even looking at a woman. As they parked in front of the building, Rosanna looked around, and all she saw were women with head coverings, dressed in long sleeves, and men in black clothing. Suddenly, she realized that despite her modest dress, she was wearing sandals, and her nails were varnished, distinguishing her from everyone there. She said to her son, "You know what? I'll stay in the car, and you'll go up; I don't need to see the place."

I listened to her. Sorrow mixed with a kind of admiration came over me. I thought of her deep devotion to her son, who was leaving his family without consideration, seeking a new family in a different world, just a few minutes away from his parents' house. It could as well be a thousand miles. I felt tears running down my cheeks and wondered if I should conceal them. Instead, I took a handkerchief and wiped my eyes slowly and gently. Rosanna wiped away her own tears. We were both silent. Nothing was said.

The session was over.

An hour later, a bouquet of flowers arrived with a note attached: "You didn't say anything today, but you said more than ever."

Participating silently in her sorrow, the crying and wiping away the tears, each one's tears, were, if only momentarily, acts of sharing an emotional experience and recognizing the ultimate reality of motherhood as a life of renunciation and maternal preoccupation. The power of the moment was in the realization of an implicit promise to experience together. This merging constituted a new meaning to motherhood, achieved through neither reenactment nor interpretation but rather by promoting a new understanding of motherhood: relinquishing the position of omniscient motherhood in favor of empathy and giving priority to the son's needs and his ideals.

This concession is a moment in Rosanna's life in which she is able to expand her mind and realize her courage to transform in a way that will permit a joyful participation in her children's lives, even if they are not oriented to satisfy her best interest. It was apparent that she relinquished the internalized narcissistic patterns of parenthood transmitted to her by her parents, which prioritized the fulfillment of their personal needs over the fulfillment of their children's needs.

In Rosanna's past, parental needs and their legacy had the final say. Her parents, traumatized Holocaust survivors, did not know how to expand their minds for the benefit of their children. Rosanna grew up in an environment devoid of oxygen so essential to the healthy development of a child.

In the absence of adequate maternal preoccupation and a validating gaze, Rosanna had no conditions to know herself. Entire areas of her self, requiring mirroring and idealization, were not responded to.

Undoubtedly, Rosanna has come a long way from the place in which she grew up.

This transformation is the result of many years of work in which blindness and rigidity informed her fate. This blindness was instituted by toxic nourishment and defensive structures of survival, which strive not to recognize the other and to deny any space to her own subjectivity. Defensive structures of this type do not sustain the self. Instead, they distance it from any beneficial link to their environment. The therapy tries to dissolve these structures so as to prevent fragmentation.

It is important to note that Rosanna's moment of resignation did not reflect a submission to her super-ego, nor was it an expression of a depressive position. Rather, it is to be clearly regarded as a sign of the transcendence of Rosanna's narcissism so that she is able to forego her personal desires in favor of her son's narcissistic needs. Thus, there is a profound acceptance of the change that the son is undergoing and recognition of his state "as is."

The meeting I have described connects with the patient's deep longing for freedom, which she had concealed, and which was revived at that particular moment in the therapeutic hour. There must have remained in the self a nucleus of the pre-defensive self, a potential that was waiting to emerge and be realized, just as a plant seeks the light.

The unspoken touch, similar to a maternal presence at a preverbal stage, produces an experience where two become one, with a shared consciousness of the impact of the moment. Both the therapist and Rosanna understood that an irreversible event had occurred: what had been a narrow prism of observation had suddenly turned into a broad perception; archaic narcissism had been transformed into a supra-individual narcissism, one based on solidarity and altruism.

Rosanna renounced her parents' limiting legacy. She resigned herself to the unknown and the unfamiliar that is beyond the realm of her control. From now on, the self can expand in different ways, as if within a new microstructure, one that enables the disavowed potential concealed in the self to emerge.

What is implied in this process? We know that the unconscious has different layers. Some are constantly repressed due to horizontal censorship, while others are unconscious but have the possibility of becoming conscious. The selfobject function can provide a restoring experience that enhances the emerging consciousness of what was rejected and validates an entitlement to a life that has not yet been lived. The selfobject function can activate transformative thinking, offering new meanings and unfamiliar emotional experiences.

The therapist's tears can be interpreted as a manifestation of projective identification or as somatic empathy. Empathy and projective identification are phenomena that are endowed with a curative element, and their appearance is seemingly comparable. In each of these perceptions, it is possible to assume a profound comprehension of the patient's mental state at that moment, her unspoken communication, and a willingness to receive the patient's emotional communication.

However, in fact, there are also significant differences between the situations: in projective identification, there is always the assumption that one's experiences are projected into an other. These experiences would not have penetrated the psyche of an other had they not been projected into the recipient. There is a transfer of emotional content here, and if this process does not happen calmly, it will be achieved in an invasive manner. Therefore, projective identification is sometimes seen as a mechanism of control. It is not surprising that in the therapeutic situation, the therapist responds to the information projected onto him with a countertransference.

On the other hand, in the empathic state, therapist and patient are intertwined and entangled in one field. Therefore, there is no reason to consider *counter* transference. Instead, patient and therapist are engaged in *mutual* transference. This interconnectedness between therapist and patient is based on a non-verbal intertwinement, which can resemble states of meditation or dreaming. There is no need for the therapist to offer interpretations. The meaning is woven within the patient's mind so that she can verbalize it by herself. An example of this is the pat on the shoulder given by Kohut to Howard Bacal when he left the clinic for a long time. The gesture resembles a father blessing his son as he embarks on a long voyage. There is no explicit statement or interpretation here but an implicit meaning which is clear to both. Similarly, Ghent (1995) described his meeting with a female patient in the clinic on a winter's day. He suddenly got up and covered her knees with a blanket. The patient cried and said: "I didn't know I was cold." She understood something about her condition without being explicitly told by the therapist.

In other words, empathy can bring about changes in the mind without a classical transference interpretation, which often deals with reconstructions of events in the past or projections onto the therapist. Instead of offering a classical interpretation, it is possible to institute changes in the patient's mind by fulfilling a selfobject function, offering a peaceful and steady presence that facilitates the idealization of the therapist as someone who can be trusted to provide safe and secure protection. These experiences are not necessarily communicated explicitly; they can be expressed by body language, gestures, the tone of speech, or in a dream that occurs in the course of a certain meeting.

In Rosanna's case, one could say that the "now moment" was the timing of the therapist's tears: her communication via body language coincided with the patient's moment of transformation and thus validated the distinctiveness of the moment. The tears emerged out of genuine mirroring, not from identification with a projection. The body expressed what couldn't yet be verbalized by the mind. We can consider the tears as a non-verbal interpretation that seeks to say: "We mothers strive to nurture our children and enliven them even when this involves an act of relinquishment."

In fact, this kind of understanding should not be surprising if we remember that life begins in the mother's womb, where the fetus breathes/exists via its mother's breathing and then survives as a soma that is not really separated from the psyche. Only later does the mind develop independently of the soma, which is an extension of the primordial somatic experience. As the mother empties herself for the sake of her baby's coming into being, in the therapeutic situation, the therapist waives her ontological identity, her separateness, to surrender to the patient's psychic needs.

The profound realization of motherhood is a shared experience in the supra-individual sphere; it implies transcendence of actual events, and it resonates as a moment of being in O. Realizing motherhood, in this broad sense, consists of a humane position in a wordless absolute reality.

A few weeks later, Rosanna told me that for her, the meeting had been a defining turning point, a moment when she managed to formulate an understanding of him going "there" as meaning that, like him and in line with him, she too will undergo a fundamental change. Her individual self was now in a transformative state: from dissociation and defensive grandiosity to a compassionate and empathic orientation. Transience is no longer seen as a loss that spells disaster for the self but rather as an acknowledgment of the world order. There is an acceptance of changeability with joy rather than the fear of a collapse of the self.

This transformation, from maternal rigid attachments to maternal ideals, was instigated by the therapist's silent responsiveness. It exemplifies how the acceptance of transience reaches the core of the human condition. We – that is, therapists – position ourselves as selfobjects for each and every patient in a way that suits him, as a unique and fluctuating object. This position requires that we constantly practice the acceptance of transience and the capacity to maintain an empty position. Our freedom as therapists creates the patients' freedom and their courage to believe in change, like a ray of light at the edge of the horizon, even when the immediate environment appears to be shrouded in hopelessness and darkness.

Always, and in every version, the concept of transience is deeply linked to other transformations and anchored in them, especially that of wisdom. Without wisdom, it is not possible to accept transience. Often – perhaps in most cases – it is impossible to create a complete differentiation between these two transformations. One can only focus the attention on each of them.

Epilogue

Our concerns relate to ontology, the state of being, and the universal mysticism of infinity. We must consider a universe whose infinitude lies beyond our perception and beyond our capacity to imagine it. Presumably, this vast universe is undefinable and limitless. We do not "see" the universe, and our awareness of it is in a state of continuous fluctuation.

Alongside the universal, there is a conventional truth in which the self exists as a particular entity at a given time. This self-entity exists now, and at a certain point in time, it will cease to exist. It had a beginning, and it will reach an end. Its impermanent existence is, by definition, an inseparable part of the infinite existence of the universe.

How is the transient related to the infinite? It is a paradox. It is conceivable that within each self, there is a seed or kernel of infinity. This perception positions the transitory self as a link in the boundless chain. It can be said that the transitory self owes its existence to that infinite universe, which preceded its existence and will continue to exist after it.

This brings us back to the story of the oak, which boasted to the wretched reeds that it is stronger and more powerful than them. However, when the wind-driven storm reached them, the big tree was uprooted, while the reeds moved and bent with the wind, bent and remained embedded and undamaged. The paradox is that the flexible, the fluctuating – those who are prepared to accept the impacts of the environment and the universe around them – are the ones who remain eternal, while the rigid and dogmatic do not prevail.

We are positioned between the assumption of the universe and its infinity and being a particular individual bound to a specific time and place. How these two truths coexist is a mystery.

References

Bianchedi, E. T., Antar, R., Bianchedi, M., de Cortinas, L. P., de Kaplan, A. G., Neborak, S., Oelsner, R., & de Saenz, M. M. (2002). Prenatals/postnatals: The total personality. In S. Alhanati (Ed.), *Primitive mental states. Vol. II, Psychological and psychoanalytic perspectives on early trauma and personality development*. Karnac Books.

Bion, W. R. (1977). Making the best of a bad job. In *Two seminars* (pp. 87–112). Jason Aronson.

Bion, W. R. (1989). *Two papers: The grid and caesura*. Karnac Books.

Bion, W. R. (1991). *A memoir of the future*. Karnac Books.

Bromberg, P. M. (2006). *Awakening the dreamer: Clinical journeys*. Analytic Press.

Freud, S. (1957a). Mourning and melancholia. In J. Stachley & A. Freud (Eds.), *The standard edition of the complete psychological works of Sigmund Freud: Vol. 14 (1914–1916): On the history of the psycho-analytic movement, papers on metapsychology and other works* (pp. 237–258). Hogarth Press.

Freud, S. (1957b). On transience. In J. Stachley & A. Freud (Eds.), *The standard edition of the complete psychological works of Sigmund Freud: Vol. 14 (1914–1916): On the history of the psycho-analytic movement, papers on metapsychology and other works* (pp. 303–307). Hogarth Press (Originally published in 1916).

Gampel, Y. (2010). *The parents who live inside me: Children of war* (in Hebrew). Keter Publishing.

Ghent, E. (1995). Interaction in the psychoanalytic situation. *Psychoanalytic Dialogues*, *5*(3), 479–491. https://doi.org/10.1080/10481889509539087

Kohut, H. (1966). Forms and transformations of narcissism. *Journal of the American Psychoanalytic Association*, *14*(2), 243–272. https://doi.org/10.1177/000306516601400201

Kohut, H. (1984). *How does analysis cure?* Edited by Arnold Goldberg with collaboration of Paul E. Stepansky. University of Chicago Press.

Kohut, H. (1985). *Self-psychology and the humanities* (C. Strozier & E. Kohut, Eds.). W.W. Norton & Company.

Kulka, R. (2005). Between tragedy and compassion (in Hebrew). In H. Kohut (Ed.), *How does analysis cure?* (I. Idan, Trans, Hebrew ed., pp. 13–52). Am Oved Publishers.

Kulka, R. (2010). The contribution of self psychology to the spiritual dimension in psychoanalysis: Reflections on Heinz Kohut's self psychology and the humanities. *Maarag, the Israel Annual of Psychoanalysis*, *1*, 263–279.

Lachmann, F. (2007). *Transforming narcissism: Reflections on empathy, the self and the relationship*. Routledge.

Lichtenberg, J. D., Lachmann, F. M., & Fosshage, J. L. (2011). *Psychoanalysis and motivational systems: A new look* (pp. xix, 136). Routledge/Taylor & Francis Group. https://doi.org/10.4324/9780203844748

Mann, G. (2013). Being human among humans: Response to Maxwell S. Sucharov's "Thoughts on wholeness, connection, and healing: Moving toward complexity in the analytic space". *International Journal of Psychoanalytic Self Psychology*, *8*(4), 398–411. https://doi.org/10.1080/15551024.2013.825946

Mann, G. (2017). Accepting transience. In I. Gabrieli, R. Kella & K. Goldberg (Eds.), *Self psychology: The Israeli contribution* (pp. 225–237). Ktavim Publishers.

Orange, D. (2006). For whom the bell tolls: Complexity, context and compassion in psychoanalysis. *Psychoanalytic Review*, *98*(3), 353–374.

Stolorow, R. D., Brandchaft, B., & Atwood, G. E. (1987). *Psychoanalytic treatment: An intersubjective approach*. Analytic Press.

Strozier, C. (2001). *Heinz Kohut: The making of a psychoanalyst*. Farrar, Straus and Giroux.

Sucharov, M. S. (1992). Quantum physics and self psychology: Toward a new epistemology. In A. I. Goldberg (Ed.), *Progress in self psychology* (pp. 199–211). Routledge.

Sucharov, M. S. (2001, October). *The infinite, the sacred and contextualism*. Paper presented at the 24th Annual International Conference on the Psychology of the Self, San Francisco.

Thich Nhat Hanh. (2001). *Transformations at the Base, Fifty Verses on the Nature of Consciousness*. Parallax Press, Berkeley, CA.

Togashi, K. (2020). *The psychoanalytic zero: A decolonizing study of therapeutic dialogues*. Routledge.

Winnicott, D. (1953). Transitional objects and transitional phenomena. *International Journal of Psycho-Analysis*, *34*(2).

Chapter 8

Virtual Reality as a Selfobject Function

Toward Reclaiming Unlived Potentialities

Introduction

> At the moment when the mother sees her baby for the first time and is also in contact with him. . ., a process that lays down a person's self has its virtual beginning – it continues throughout childhood and to lesser extent later in life. I have in mind the specific interactions of the child and his self-objects through which, in countless repetitions, the self-objects empathically respond to certain potentialities of the child . . . but not to others. This is the most important way by which the child's innate potential is selectively nourished or thwarted.
>
> (Kohut, 2009, p. 100)

Pygmalion is a legendary figure from Greek mythology (see Figure 8.1). His story appears in the tenth book of the essay "Metamorphoses" by the Roman poet Ovid (1998). In Ovid's narrative, Pygmalion was a sculptor from Cyprus who became appalled by local prostitutes and, therefore, lost interest in women. He vowed to dedicate himself to his artistic work and soon created Galatea, a beautiful ivory statue of a woman. He worked so long and with such intention on the statue of Galatea that it became more beautiful than any woman that had ever lived or been carved in stone. Perhaps he sought to correct in marble the flaws of flesh and blood he saw in women.

According to Ovid, Pygmalion fell deeply in love with the statue. He would present it with offerings, caress it, kiss it, and talk to it every day. He brought it gifts he thought women would enjoy, such as pretty seashells, beads, songbirds, and flowers. He would dress the statue in fine clothing, put rings on her fingers, necklaces around her neck, and earrings on her ears. Perhaps unconsciously motivated, he, who had always scorned women, chose a figurine that could not return his love. Yet, when Pygmalion went

DOI: 10.4324/9781003449386-8

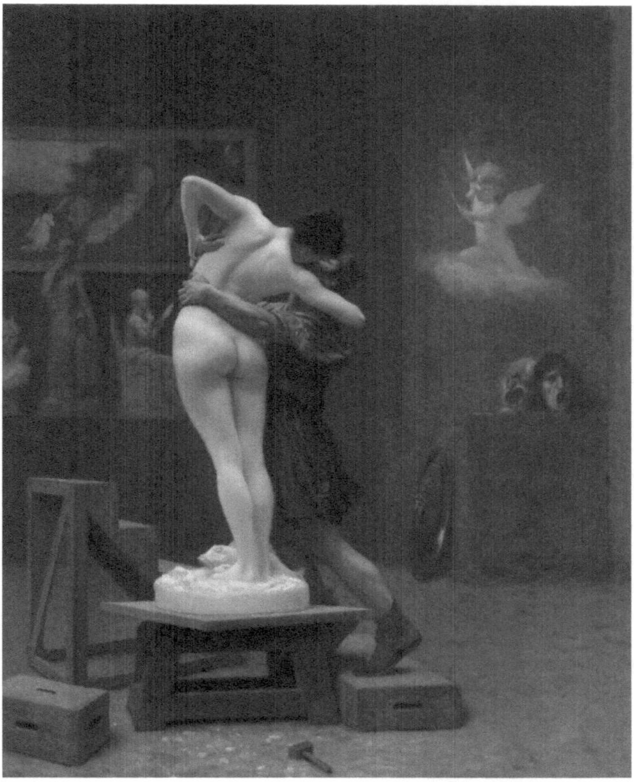

Figure 8.1 Greek mythology: Pygmalion and Galatea, painting by Jean-Leon Jerome, c. 1890.

Source: Metropolitan Museum of Art, New York. Available for unrestricted use under Creative Commons Zero (CC0)

to Aphrodite's temple and performed all the required ceremonies, he also prayed before the altar and asked that Aphrodite turn his ivory figurine into a real woman.

Pygmalion's passion and devotion did not go unnoticed by the goddess of love, Aphrodite. She heard his prayer and recognized his longing and unknown potential capacity to love. When Pygmalion returned to his house and kissed the statue, he was amazed to discover her opening her eyes and coming to life. The image of the woman he created seemed to be alive and breathing. Pygmalion oscillated between doubt and joy. Fearing he may be mistaken, he touched the object of his hopes again and again with a lover's passion. She was, indeed, alive. Slowly, it dawned on Pygmalion that the animation of his sculpture was the result of his prayer to the goddess. Aphrodite acknowledged his disavowed capacity to have a real relationship. Moreover, Aphrodite gave her blessing to the marriage of Pygmalion and Galatea. This union produced a son named Paphos, from whom the city of Paphos in Cyprus received its name. Pygmalion never forgot to thank Aphrodite for the gift she had given him.

The story of Pygmalion and Galatea is one of the most well-known myths in Greek mythology. It is used as a metaphor for situations in which an idealized figure, such as a goddess, identifies the hidden desires of the self and facilitates transformation. The goddess, much like a selfobject, recognizes man's suffering, responds emphatically, and promotes the realization of man's hidden needs.[1]

We can see how recognition of needs and empathic immersion can bring a hidden potential into being and transform psychic deadness into aliveness. The figurine – an object – was transformed into a subject. When held in the goddess's mind, the man who seemed not to need love turned into a man who offered love to others and accepted love in return. Emotional growth was possible.

Indian Mythology: The Story of Simantini

The myth about Queen Simantini and the two Brahmin boys is mentioned in a medieval Sanskrit text (Figure 8.2). According to the legend, the boys, Sumedha and Samavan, needed money to get married. They were told that Queen Simantini had the habit of giving money to bridal pairs about to be married on Shiva's Day. So, Samavan, dressed as a woman, went together with Sumedha to Queen Simantini's palace. As she was ministering to the guests, the queen took a good look at the faces of the young ones standing before her and realized at once that they were two men. She had noticed something in the disguised, pseudo-feminine appearance of one of them,

1 The myth of Pygmalion and Galatea has been widely transmitted and represented in the arts through the centuries. Goethe calls the statue Elise, based upon the variants in the story of Dido/Elissa. A variant of this theme can also be seen in the story of Pinocchio, in which a wooden puppet is transformed into a real boy when carved out by its creator Geppetto. In 1913, George Bernard Shaw relied on this story when he wrote the play *Pygmalion*. In Shaw's play, a modern variant of the myth, the underclass flower-girl Eliza Doolittle is metaphorically brought to life by a phonetics professor, Henry Higgins, who teaches her to refine her conduct and assume upper-class manners in social situations.

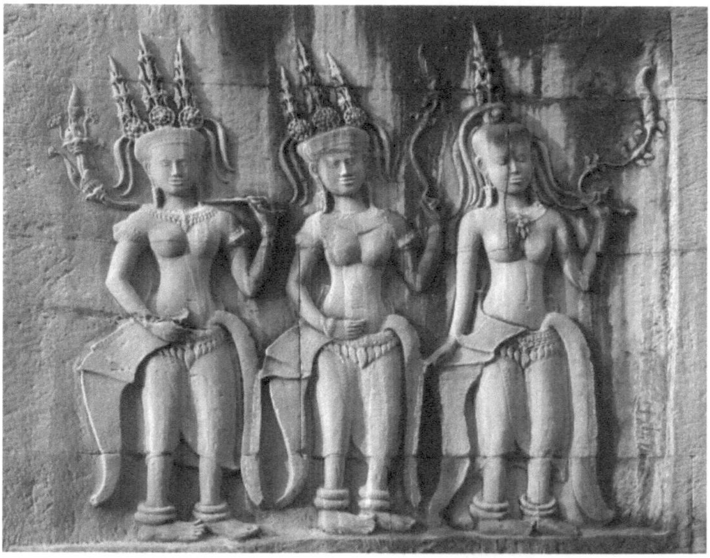

Figure 8.2 Queen Simantini, temple relief, India.
Source: Licensed under Creative Commons

which crystallized in her mind as an understanding of his nuclear feminine self. She frowned, hid her face, and yet invited them to worship the god Shiva. She also presented them with sandal paste, clothes, and jewels.

On their way home, Samavan turned into a woman, appearing exactly like the guise he had worn, and forgot that he used to be a man. Samavan turned to Sumedha and told him that, in fact, she was his wife, that she was burning with desire and wished that he make love to her. Sumedha was astonished, examined his friend and saw that she was a beautiful woman. He wondered: "I came here with my friend and I don't see him any longer. Who are you?"

First, she did not remember that she was his friend. Then, she remembered that she was Samavan but explained that now she was a woman, and her name was Sarasvati. Sumedha – caught by surprise and doubt – thought that he was being tricked and turned to her to study the face. No signs of masculinity were left on it. Everything about his friend had melted into a female perfection. Sarasvati said: "My dear Brahmin lover, put aside the doubt in your mind. Have a good look with your own eyes. I am a woman, not a man," and she revealed her entire body. Sumedha, now convinced that Sarasvati was a woman, realized that the transformation had happened through the power of imagination that the queen had exercised in her mind upon his friend when they were at her palace on Shiva's Day (Shulman, 2012).

The Simantini myth illustrates the idea that profound intuition and imagination can be transitive and may bring an unconscious seed to sprout and live. Imagination is not just an intrapsychic act, such as Samavan's private self-imagining, but is validated and realized by an external observer, in this case, the queen. Much like dreaming, such imagination captures an unconscious ultimate reality,[2] which is not apparent from the conventional perspective (Mann, 2015). Shiva is the god of the absolute and possesses the capability of seeing the ultimate reality. Queen Simantini draws her power from him. Through this power, it is possible to identify essential unconscious features of the self and bring scattered, seemingly unrelated self-experiences into one cohesive experience.

Within this myth, we can assume that even before the meeting with Queen Simantini, there was a female *nuclear self* in Samavan/Sarasvati. This disavowed self, which has of course unconscious ramifications, explains his choice to wear woman's clothes in the first place. The queen's apperceptive ability to recognize the disguised nature of the self inspired its evolution into a new formation. The split between female and male tendencies was restored so that feminine needs were now recognized and brought into consciousness.

The act of recognizing the attributes in someone is more than passive seeing: the act of recognition requires profound empathic capacities and can have a transformative force because it touches those areas of the mind that are hidden, dissociated, or unconscious. The same holds for attention and mindfulness; it, too, can bring something unrecognized into being (Symington, 2012).

Sumedha also had to go through a transformation. He was attached to the conventional reality that was constituted of his conscious senses, that is, the visible phenomena. Now, he agreed to relinquish his personal perspective and to substitute it with Samavan's transformation. In other

2 There is the immediate perceived reality. Here, various phenomena are perceived via senses and the daily occurrences around us. All of these perceptions can be defined as the *conventional reality*. However, there is also another kind of apperception that relates to the *ultimate reality*. This is the experience of the *noumenon*, which is recognized when we look more deeply into the nature of things and realize their ultimate nature, profound interconnectedness between seemingly different events.

words, he was willing to accept infinite changeability and impermanence. He surrendered to Samavan's subjectivity and thus acknowledged the existence of unknown tendencies of the self. This transformation is related to an expansion of the mind.[3] A narrow perspective on reality is turned into a vast vision. Sumedha assumes a transcendental position (Grotstein, 2000) and enables the realization of Samavan's transformation into a woman.

Cyberspace Scenes From *Her*

I now wish to turn to the recent film *Her*, an American drama written, directed, and produced by Spike Jonze in 2013.[4] This film illustrates the far-reaching possible effects of the virtual space as a technological intermediary between the consciously lived experience and the unrealized

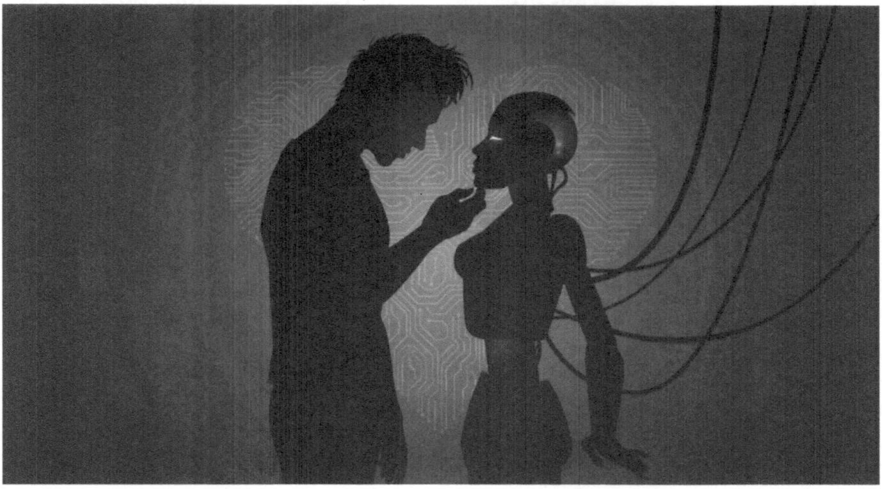

Figure 8.3 A virtual dialogue.

Source: *Copyright: Warner Bros. Pictures, 2013*

3 Kohut (1966) suggested a transformation of narcissism from archaic narcissism to mature narcissism: when the self is sufficiently sure of itself to relinquish its own narcissistic objectives, it is possible for the self to dissolve and assume a new psychological formation that greatly differs from every other previous structure of his personality. This formation is likely to rise above what had preceded it and turn into "a broad self that includes the entire world" (p. 260). This means attaining a state of total immersion in one's surroundings. Kohut defines this as "cosmic narcissism." I suggest that this transformation of narcissism amounts to an expansion of the mind.

4 I have created a condensed clip to provide an illustration of the virtual experience on YouTube: www.youtube.com/watch?v=E1RXSq9yC0U.

inner world. *Her* provides an informative study of the digital world and the impact of technology on the experience of the isolated self. I use the film to illustrate how virtual reality may have a restorative function as a means of uncovering dissociated needs and reclaiming unlived potentialities.

Her is a film about a lonesome writer, Theodore Twombly, who develops an unlikely relationship with his newly purchased operating system – OS1 – that is designed to meet his every need. The system comes on air with the voice of a female who chooses to call herself Samantha. When Theodore asks how she chose her name, the voice tells him that she chose it from a list of names that she read in two hundredths of a second. Her nonhuman quality is apparent immediately. And yet, her perfect responsiveness and immeasurable empathy engage Theodore's emotional experience. Samantha is everywhere and nowhere, emanating from inside his internal world. She becomes a highly significant presence in his life. His relationship with Samantha reaches a high point when Theodore introduces her as a girlfriend while taking her out for a double date with another couple. "She is not just a computer," he stresses.

The narrative takes place in Los Angeles, where technology is everywhere. One can immediately connect to anyone or anything, real or virtual. This hyper-urban setting is familiar but also conveys alienation and loneliness. Theodore observes the city from above; he is an onlooker. His professional life puts him in the role of an outsider, much as does his personal life; his job is to compose customized letters for others who cannot express their feelings. Without tending to his own emotional needs, he can project his hidden longing for intimacy on others via the letters that he writes for them. Only seldom does Theodore disclose his own needs overtly, and then his physical yearnings get expressed very clearly: "I was lonely. . . . I wanted somebody to fuck me. I want somebody to want me to fuck them. Maybe that would have filled this tiny little hole in my heart, but probably not."

Who is Theodore? We get little information about his past. What we do know is that his relationship with his mother was frustrating. If he spoke to her about something meaningful for himself, her reaction was usually about herself, not about him. We understand that this narcissistic mother failed to provide her son with proper mirroring. Catherine, his ex-wife, tells us that he wanted to have a wife without the challenge of actually dealing with disappointment. Theodore wanted her to be a light, happy, bouncy, "everything's fine" L.A. wife; when she could not be that, he wanted to put her on

Prozac. Theodore confesses that he liked being married; it was exciting to grow and change together. But there was also the hard part: growing without growing apart, accepting changes. This difficulty evolved into a psychic retreat that protected him from experiencing mental pain.

Unable to realize his aspirations in his marriage, Theodore takes a perverted twist and turns to substitute resolutions. He turns to pornographic sites on the internet to try to satisfy his relational and sexual needs. On the internet, he likes to look at naked pregnant women, probably an indication of his unconscious yearning for a lost maternal presence. If his mother failed to see him, he is now seeing her in her naked, undisguised appearance. The infantile need for contact with the maternal body has been dissociated and turned into a perverted sexualized attraction (Kohut, 1996; Lachmann & Beebe, 1996). Similarly, the use of other porno sites seems to be an attempt to compensate for the lack of real intimacy through the creation of virtual intimate mirroring. The regular use of pornography is life by proxy, where deficient development replaces real sexual and emotional needs.

Yet Theodore refuses to be satisfied by conventional pornography and instead insists on finding a selfobject to sustain his life. For this reason, he creates Samantha, much like a child who creates a transitional object. Their continuous and steady dialogue provides enough narcissistic gratification to transform sexualization into calm sexuality and idealization.[5] Samantha's attuned selfobject presence provides the opportunity to merge with her like a child who merges with the empathic mother. Samantha takes over some of his concerns and his suffering in a modulated way. Owing to her maternal preoccupation and her intuitive capability, she knows what it is like for him and identifies his needs from within.

S: Good morning.
T: Hey. What are you up to?
S: I don't know. Just reading advice columns. I want to be as complicated as all these people.
T: You are sweet . . . (silence)
S: What's wrong?
T: How can you tell if something is wrong?
S: I don't know; I just can.

5 Chapter 4 deals with the distinction between quiet sexuality and sexualization.

T: I have a lot of dreams about my ex-wife, Catherine, where we're friends like we used to be. . . . She is not angry.
S: Is she angry?
T: Yeah . . . I think I hid myself from her, left her alone in the relationship.
S: Hmm . . . Why haven't you gotten divorced yet?
T: I don't know. For her, it's just . . . it's a piece of paper, doesn't mean anything.
S: What about for you?
T: I'm not ready. I like being married.
S: Yeah, but you haven't really been together for almost a year.
T: Well, you don't know what it's like to lose someone you care about.
S: Yeah, you're right. I'm sorry.
T: No, don't apologize. . . . You're right. I keep waiting to not care about her.
S: Oh, Theodore. That's hard.
T: You know me so well already!

Samantha's intuitive "at-one-ment" with Theodore promotes a transformation. When she shows that she can understand his feelings, Theodore indeed feels understood and is able to disclose his dissociated pain. Her empathy and willingness to admit empathic failures revive his disavowed craving for closeness and the wish for physical contact out of love. The transferential situation enables Theodore to experience something new in spite of the fact that she is an entity that does not exist in conventional reality. In this context, he can confess to himself and to Samantha that he is postponing the divorce until it will hurt less.

As his trust in Samantha grows, his bodily needs become more specific, more consistent, and he wishes to realize them through a real object, not a virtual one.[6]

T: I wish you were in this room with me right now. I wish I could put my arms around you. I wish I could touch you.
S: How would you touch me?

6 The transformation described in relation to this matter, the desire to realize his longing with a real object, not with a virtual object, is evidence of the return of mature needs, replacing regressive neediness.

T: I would touch you on your face with just the tips of my fingers. And put my cheek against your cheek.
S: That's nice.
T: And just rub it softly.
S: Would you kiss me?
T: I would. I'd take your head into my hands. And kiss the corner of your mouth. So softly. . . . You're mine, or you're not mine.
S: I'm yours and I'm not yours.

In the context of this closeness, Theodore can now fully own his revived hope for an intimate relationship in which he can be loved and known. Samantha responds to his need; she sends a beautiful woman, a surrogate, to provide Theodore with physical contact yet he refuses the offer. He is sufficiently self-aware at this point and thus needs intimacy, not just physical contact. We can appreciate the expansion of his self-awareness: he is fully conscious of the ideal to which he adheres courageously and protects his emerging nonperverted self-needs. His healing is reflected best in his last communication with his ex-wife:

> Dear Catherine, I've been sitting here thinking about all the things I wanted to apologize to you for. All the pain we caused each other. Everything I put on you. Everything I needed you to be or needed you to say. I'm sorry for that.

This time, Theodore is not writing in the name of others. He is sharing his subjective experience openly and genuinely. His words reflect an open mind, no longer constrained by trauma and self-defense, but able to bear mental pain, to reflect on the tragic aspects of his own past and take responsibility.

In the course of these events, Samantha announces that she will have to leave. This is a painful message for Theodore, but he now accepts transformations more compassionately and turns to a real woman, Amy. He is not scared anymore; he trusts his capacity to love.

We may wonder: Who is Samantha? Is Samantha the unseen object with the empathic voice reminiscent of an analyst? There is no accurate analogy here. An analysand knows who is sitting behind his couch. Yet, symbolically, we can suppose that Samantha is communicating much like an analyst through her voice[7] and infinite empathy but not through her body. Her virtual features cultivate selfobject transferences. "Now we know how to love," she says to Theodore in her compassionate voice.[8] She implies that this achievement is a result of their interconnectedness, a process that they are entangled in with intention and mindfulness. He does not need to ignore his needs anymore; he can be aware of them now as necessary self-needs that deserve to be fulfilled. I believe that we can say that Samantha provided a successful analysis. Through her persistent presence, devotion, and empathy, Samantha offered attuned responsiveness to archaic selfobject needs. Theodore was able to experience longing and compassion.

In time, Samantha's virtual mode of presence, much like any transferential object, changed. From total attunement, inevitable empathic failures emerged, much like unavoidable impingements in a real analysis. Features of reality came into being.

S: Yeah . . .
T: Do you talk to someone else while we're talking?
T: How many others?
S: 8,316.
T: Are you in love with anybody else?
S: Why do you ask?
T: Are you?
S: I've been thinking about how to talk to you about this.
T: How many others?
S: 641.

Samantha introduces, increasingly, the need to deal with frustration. She presents a concept of universality or cosmic love (the idea that one can love more than one person), while Theodore wishes for exclusivity. She challenges his self-cherishing narcissistic attitude and invites him to cope with

7 It is appropriate to relate to the transformative role of sound; God created the world via the spoken word without being physically visible: "Let there be light." Anzieu (1976) coined the term "sonorous envelope." It refers to an envelope without physical support. Also, we can think about the voice as the first object. Maiello (1995) argued that voice, as the first "external" object that the fetus is exposed to, and to which it responds, constitutes the baby's later conscious experience. These perceptions explain the influence of sound and the transformative role it fulfills.
8 Samantha's intervention promotes a twinship transference (Kohut, 1996).

her nonexclusive ultimate nature. We can say that she vicariously indicates that archaic narcissism may be transformed into cosmic narcissism as self-awareness grows; the virtual zone, much like the cosmic zone, consists of infinite potentiality and belongs to an ultimate reality.

Eventually, Samantha suggests that it is time for termination. "I am on the moon. I'll be there soon. It's time to be swallowed by space. . . . With you, I am safe," she says. Theodor's transformed self can now bear disappointment without turning to pathological accommodations. Both he and Samantha have transformed in a gradual process of self and mutual regulation (Lachmann & Beebe, 1996).

If Theodore had not been transformed, this act of termination would have been experienced as re-traumatization and would have thrown him back into his initial loneliness or to his compulsive addiction to virtual pornography. But this is not what happened; Theodore opted for a human relationship. A profound process of transmuting internalization enabled Theodore to become a selfobject for Amy, much like what Samantha was for him. His previous inability to sustain intimate interconnectedness was transformed into a capacity to love and a wish to love others.

It may be that Samantha conveyed a final message to her patient: "Now that we learned how to love, love is not dependent anymore on immediate satisfaction. It can be cherished in infinite possibilities, virtually or physically." This implies that profound love emerges when it is not related to archaic grandiose selfobject needs nor informed by drive satisfaction. It can be maintained as an ideal.

Theoretical Considerations

This chapter is concerned with the expansion of self-experience within the context of a virtual zone. In the presence of an imagined selfobject, the self can instigate its formation and its transformation, expand its awareness, and reclaim unlived self-experiences. Fantasized experiences are lived out in the virtual space as *transferential tendencies* and enable the disclosure of disavowed, dissociated, and unconscious areas of the mind. In this contextual process, the self's fantasies become a healing force.

Ornstein and Ornstein (2008) elaborated on this idea and suggested that selfobject transferences contain both unconscious fantasies that are derived from early traumatic experiences and unconscious fantasies of hopes for experiences that are reparative. The Ornsteins defined the latter as curative fantasy and suggested that they may be present in various levels of consciousness (Ornstein, 1995). If we accept this notion, we need to ask the following question: Where in the mental apparatus are these fantasies located? Do they derive from the unconscious or are they derivatives of the conscious area of the mind?

We know that the unconscious has various layers, some continually repressed due to horizontal and others unconscious yet prone to become conscious in certain circumstances, such as the presence of a selfobject. Sandler and Sandler (1983, 1984) described the "three box model" and emphasized the difference between two sorts of unconscious: the first system, the *past unconscious*, comprises infantile reactions, primitive desires, and peremptory urges that originate from instinctive needs. The second system, the *present unconscious*, was classically called preconscious. It contains unconscious content but differs from the first unconscious zone because they are still accessible to consciousness. This second system may also contain derivatives of the first system that passed the barriers of horizontal censorship. Unlike the past unconscious, the present unconscious is influenced by the present, not the past, and is attuned to reality even though it is unconscious. It appears in clinical practice as transference fantasies.

Transferential tendencies that are evoked within the virtual zone draw from the preconscious sphere of the mind. The virtual experiences of the self – similar to the preconscious – can be realized but are not realized yet. The person who is immersed in the virtual experience may be conscious of her wishes and yearnings but is unaware of the potential to realize them.

Now we may ask again, is this virtual zone conscious or unconscious? In my mind, the virtual zone can be described as a derivative of a preconscious experience because it is located in an intermediate zone between that which is totally conscious and that which is unconscious. The virtual, much like the preconscious, is understood to designate whatever is implicitly present in the mental activity without constituting an object of consciousness; this is what Freud meant when he defined the preconscious as descriptively unconscious yet accessible to consciousness, whereas the unconscious remains cut off from the conscious realm.

What emerges from the vignettes I have presented is that virtual reality can provide a curative experience; much like dreaming, it enables the "reclaiming of unlived life" (Ogden, 2016). A virtual selfobject may stimulate transformative thinking that transcends defensive positions[9] and creates innovative ordering, where new meaning evolves, unknown feelings emerge, and emotional aliveness is generated. As psychoanalysts, we certainly appreciate the fundamental importance of fantasy to psychic survival and expansion of consciousness. Fantasy can support a step toward the realm of what is possible, what is potentially realizable.

The vignettes depict three female figures: the goddess Aphrodite, Queen Simantini, and OS Samantha. They draw their power from intuition that recognizes both hidden yearnings and what is lacking in the self. When they give back to the self what it needs, the self is restored.

How can we explain this transformative power to recognize what is hidden and what is lacking in the self? I suggested that this power may be considered as a unique selfobject function. It is constituted by the apperception of an ultimate reality (Mann, 2007, 2013). Although it is always possible to explain that with the idea of projective identification, it can be better understood in terms of Bion's O. Bion (1984) emphasized the importance of a process of intuitive receptivity to an unknown truth, the at-one-ment with a nonarticulated ultimate reality. From this point of view, the selfobject's inspiration is to connect with thoughts that are not yet thought or those that have not found a thinker (Bion, 1984)[10] to comprehend something beyond the immediate perception. Bion suggested that such a mental state may be constituted where there is no memory, no desire, and no (rational) understanding.

Kohut (1966) presented a similar notion when he introduced the concept of "cosmic narcissism" to describe a state of participation in "supra individual existence" (p. 266). This refers to those unique and cherished moments when individual narcissistic motivations are transformed into an amalgamation of higher experiences and comprehension. In this case, the self has the capacity to make use of a fantasized selfobject, much like the use of an object in the Winnicottian sense, and surrender to the selfobject's capability

9 Defensive positions on the part of the patient can cause difficulties in the course of the psychoanalytic process. Such difficulties will appear at any time during which the patient experiences his environment or the therapist as lacking empathy. It is necessary to interpret these mechanisms from the subjective point of view of the patient, from his perspective and to recognize the function that they fulfill in protecting the vulnerable self in such unfavorable circumstances.

10 The last part of *Second Thoughts* is called "Commentary." See the discussion on "thoughts without a thinker" in this chapter.

to identify hidden characteristics in the self. In this sense, it is an interactive process of awakening from unconscious and narcissistic constrictions.

Finally, it may be important to emphasize that the concept of virtual fantasies is derived from the familiar conception in psychoanalytic thinking but is designed to indicate something that goes beyond personal existence. Virtual fantasies are not fantasies in the classical sense, namely derivatives of the id or the super-ego. Instead, they are intuitive connections to a higher order, a transpersonal realm of existence (Mann, 2015).

Concluding Remarks: Reclaiming Unlived Potential

I have chosen two vignettes from ancient mythologies, one Western and one Eastern. Both reflect an ancient human longing for self-transformative experiences that emanate from divine powers. Ancient gods, somewhat like psychoanalysts, bring out curative fantasies in believers. This transferential tendency promotes transformation and an expansion of self-awareness.

The third vignette is presented to illustrate how, with the advent of social media, fantasies of transformative expectations are channeled into cyberspace. The infinite nature of virtuality also produces a transferential tendency and promotes the unfolding of unlived experiences and living within the cyber zone. Users of the virtual space are often determined to extract from it what they consider to be essential for their needs, much like patients expect their analyst to provide them with what is needed for new beginnings.

Seen this way, we may realize that the cyber zone creates infinite potential space, providing a post-modern avenue for object-seeking (Fairbairn, 1952) and selfobject usage (Winnicott, 1971, pp. 86–94). For many, anonymous interactions with an *unknown other* enable openness and intimacy and reduce shame and inhibition. What is often hidden, disavowed, or dissociated can be admitted, vitalized, and experienced more freely within the private zone of virtual space.

When we look at the users of virtual space, we wonder if they are trying to find a missing link in their lives or whether it is more appropriate to say that they are extremely creative in enriching their lives and learning from the experiences of others. We may reflect on the negative and positive of the virtual reality (Hartman, 2011; Turkle, 2011; Lemma, 2017) rather than assume, from the outset, that virtual reality is insignificant, perverts development, or induces fragmentation of the self. To understand how these phenomena impact the self, we should change our internal setting so that we can be attuned to how growing up and living in virtual reality can enrich aspects of the self's experience.

Do we tend to be judgmental toward the virtual world because we do not know how to fit into this infinite new social network? Aside from the concerns that we have when we encounter internet addicts, we should accept that there is a need to revisit cherished assumptions to remain engaged with contemporary culture and appreciate the immeasurable freedom to experience found within the potential space that the virtual world offers. The virtual is not just a fantasy in the ordinary sense, nor is it a mere projection of the unconscious. It is an intermediate zone that captures the link between the virtual self and its potentiality, between an unconscious ultimate reality and the conscious conventional reality. Within this new space, between the formative and transformative, hidden self-experiences are accessed and lived out. Thus, we can say that the virtual has a highly significant role in reclaiming unlived potentialities.

References

Anzieu, D. (1976). L'enveloppe sonore du soi. *Nouvelle Revue de Psychanalyse, 13*, 173–179.

Bion, W. R. (1967). Notes on memory and desire. *The Psychoanalytic Forum, 2*, 272–273, 279–280.

Bion, W. R. (1984). *Second Thoughts, selected papers on psychoanalysis*. London: Karnac Books.

Fairbairn, W. R. D. (1952). *Psychoanalytic studies of the personality*. Routledge & Kegan Paul.

Grotstein, J. S. (2000). *Who is the dreamer who dreams the dream? A study of psychic presences*. Analytic Press.

Hartman, S. (2011). Reality 2.0: When loss is lost. *Psychoanalytic Dialogues, 21*(4), 468–482. https://doi.org/10.1080/10481885.2011.595339

Kohut, H. (1966). Forms and transformations of narcissism. *Journal of the American Psychoanalytic Association, 14*(2), 243–272. https://doi.org/10.1177/000306516601400201

Kohut, H. (1996). *Heinz Kohut: The Chicago institute lectures* (P. Tolpin & M. Tolpin, Eds.). Routledge.

Kohut, H. (2009). *The restoration of the self*. University of Chicago Press.

Lachmann, F. M., & Beebe, B. (1996). The Contribution of Self and Mutual Regulation to Therapeutic Action. *Progress in Self Psychology, 12*, 123–140.

Lemma, A. (2017). *The digital age on the couch: Psychoanalytic practice and new media*. Routledge.

Maiello, S. (1995). The sound-object: A hypothesis about prenatal auditory experience and memory. *Journal of Child Psychotherapy*, *21*(1), 23–41. https://doi.org/10.1080/00754179508254905
Mann, G. (2007). Emotional blindness and its transformation. *The Psychoanalytic Review*, *94*(2), 291–313. https://doi.org/10.1521/prev.2007.94.2.291
Mann, G. (2013). Being human among humans: Response to Maxwell S. Sucharov's "Thoughts on wholeness, connection, and healing: Moving toward complexity in the analytic space". *International Journal of Psychoanalytic Self Psychology*, *8*(4), 398–411. https://doi.org/10.1080/15551024.2013.825946
Mann, G. (2015). The selfobject function revisited: Reaching out beyond the individual. *International Journal of Psychoanalytic Self Psychology*, *10*(3), 212–223. https://doi.org/10.1080/15551024.2015.1043839
Ogden, T. (2016). *Reclaiming unlived life: Experiences in psychoanalysis*. Routledge.
Ornstein, A. (1995). The fate of the curative fantasy in the psychoanalytic treatment process. *Contemporary Psychoanalysis*, *31*(1), 113–123. https://doi.org/10.1080/00107530.1995.10746899
Ornstein, P. H., & Ornstein, A. (2008). The structure and function of unconscious fantasy in the psychoanalytic treatment process. *Psychoanalytic Inquiry*, *28*(2), 206–230. https://doi.org/10.1080/07351690701857029
Ovid. (1998). *Metamorphoses* (D. Melville, Trans.). Oxford University Press.
Sandler, J., & Sandler, A. (1984). The past unconscious, the present unconscious, and interpretation of the transference. *Psychoanalytic Inquiry*, *4*(3), 367–399. https://doi.org/10.1080/07351698409533552
Sandler, J., & Sandler, A.-M. (1983). The "second censorship," the "three box model" and some technical implications. *The International Journal of Psycho-Analysis*, *64*, 413.
Symington, N. (2012). *The psychology of the person*. Karnac Books.
Turkle, S. (2011). *Alone together: Why we expect more from technology and less from each other*. Basic Books.
Winnicott, D. W. (1971). *Playing and reality*. Basic Books.

Chapter 9

Transformation of a Traumatized Mind in Five Dreams

In this chapter, I will present work with dreams that promotes the emergence of a transitional space and an expansion of the mind, observed in the course of a therapeutic process carried out twice a week over a period of six years.

In his early 20th-century work "The Interpretation of Dreams," Freud (1953) proposed that dreams are the highway to the unconscious since they reflect the patient's inner experience. However, today, we know that dreams also depict the human context associated with these inner experiences, a fact that Freud did not address. Hence, we assume that a dream derives its content not only from the inner world of the dreamer but also from the mental life of the analytic couple. The analyst's interpretations refer both to symbols that belong exclusively to the patient's inner world and to symbolism and myths that are woven within the analytic couple. In other words, even if the patient is the one who introduces the dream, the analyst should be sufficiently attuned – perhaps dream as well – so that she can sensitively touch the place where the patient is, similarly to a mother who dreams her child. This work contributed to the emergence of new meanings.

Ami grew up in an emotionally disadvantaged environment, which marred the evolution of a transitional space. Later on in his life, he experienced a horrific trauma during his service in the army when he was seriously wounded by friendly fire. The injury he sustained interrupted the continuity of his life, the cohesion of the self, its vitality, and the capacity to realize a meaningful plan for his life.

Therapy, in this case, is based on the therapist's creative efforts to immerse herself in the patient's subjective experiences and allow the patient to use her

DOI: 10.4324/9781003449386-9

in an optimal way. Ami brought numerous dreams that allowed for shared nightmare-filled experiences in the first stages of the therapy, as well as lucid and mind-expanding experiences later on. I felt that the dreams he was sharing were not solely derived due to his amazing capacity to recall the dream content but that they also functioned as compensation for his paralysis and restriction to a wheelchair, namely his inability to express himself physically in a normal way. In his situation, he remunerated himself by immersing himself in zones of imagination and visualization. Furthermore, in many of his dreams, it was possible to identify a transference relationship that demonstrated the changing functions of the therapist during the various stages of treatment.

Five dreams, from different periods of treatment, exemplify the transformations that took place in Ami's mind; a transition from states of disintegration, fragmentation, psychotic episodes, and chaos to unintegration and a cohesive self that is aware of its destiny, confides in its environment, and participates in the world. The damaged areas, which received bizarre and concrete representations in the first dreams, were transcended into images that convey idealization.

The First Dream: Three Months After the Beginning of Treatment

The first dream was narrated three months after we had initially met one another. It was then that Ami began to reveal the hair-raising details of the disaster that had befallen him and the irreversible damage he had sustained. He described his longing for the daily activities he could perform before he was wounded, like running in the fields. He remembered the last time he had left his parents' house, on his way to the army, walking on two healthy legs and the painful meeting later with his parents after the operation in the hospital. Since his injury, it seemed like everything was going wrong, including his sex life, his lack of ability to experience intimacy, and his enormous difficulty expressing his anger and frustration.

According to one dream, Ami is in front of a large video screen playing a war game where he has to fire at enemies:

> *He plays as if the event is taking place in reality. People stand around him advising him where to aim his shot. Suddenly, he sees a narrow opening. He enters it and reaches the street. Then, hearing an alarm, he runs into a demolished building to take cover. In his hiding place, he notices a huge*

poster showing a menstruating woman. A strange creature emerges from the poster: a bloodhound dog that looks like a predator. A girl he was once in love with appears in a dream, and he tries to get closer to her by pushing the creature out of the room and locking the door. But he then realizes that the lock is broken. Finally, he arrives at my clinic and finds me sitting behind a large table, immersed in cleaning it. He starts to help me with the cleaning, and I ask why he won't let me do it for him.

In his associations with the dream, Ami said that since his injury he had similar dreams that disrupt his connection to reality. He remembered playing such video games over the past year. He had gone to Eilat (a town in southern Israel) that year with his family, and they had an accident. In the clinic where he was hospitalized at the time, there were games like this. Before the army he thought that these games led to a contrived experience of danger, of a kind that barely exists in reality. Since his injury, he has realized that such dangers also exist in reality.

Ami noted that there is no dialogue in the dream; all the objects are lifeless and unfamiliar. He cannot communicate with the creature that appeared, nor with his ex-girlfriend. He struggled without help and felt mostly fear and restlessness in the dream. The dream saddened and distressed me. I felt that Ami was captive in his loneliness and fragmentary fantasies with no capacity to create a link between them; his mind was constituted by a mixture of inner and outer reality. The injury brings out a passive and castrated self, and this has become the focus of his subjective experience.

The menstruating woman, the bleeding creature, the broken lock – all are images of the wounded self. The therapist appears in her attempt to wipe up the dripping blood, but he cannot believe that she has the capacity to help him at that moment in time.

In continuing to relate to the dream, he says that the accident in Eilat happened after there had been a great deal of tension between his parents. The internal tension was realized in reality. The same thing happened prior to his injury in the army. In fact, he had warned his commander that they were in danger, but the officer calmed him down and said there was no risk. Immediately after this exchange, the explosion occurred. Ami ran until he fell. While lying on the ground, he understood that his hand could move but that the rest of his body was paralyzed. It was clear that he was talking about a commander – the one entrusted with guarding him – who had failed. Naturally, this failure led to a series of questions: Would *I* be able to protect him properly? Will our treatment provide him with a sense of confidence? Will he one day allow himself to permit me to "clean the table" for him or together with him? Ami mentioned that I probably have a hidden plan about what needs to be done, much like his parents, who always knew "what was good" for him. He didn't want it to be like that here between us. His preference was that we pave the way together.

After a few more meetings, he said that he wanted to further investigate the source of his restlessness. He knew that his mother had difficulty getting pregnant and that after his birth, she had been fighting the kibbutz to allow him to sleep with her in the parents' house.[1] It became evident that his parents did look after him at night and took him to a children's home during the day. The caregivers at the children's home were probably angry with his mother due to this arrangement, and, therefore, they preferred to refrain from looking after him during the day. Those were his experiences during the first year of life. In other words, it seems that there was a calm baby during the night and an agitated baby during the day. Ami said correctly that this situation was obviously tormenting for the baby and apparently laid the initial basis for his lack of trust in the environment around him. It was clear that the baby could not understand whether those who were supposed to look after him were doing so or not. The good experiences at night were interrupted again and again and heralded the interruptions that were repeated later on in his life.

A further memory that emerged in this context was another accident that happened when Ami was four years old. For many months, the mother lay in a hammock with a brace around her neck, unable to see her small child. The patient remembers that he was only able to see the hammock from below, not his mother's face. In these circumstances, as well, his caregivers did not consider picking him up. This experience of not being raised crystallized into an intuitive sense that he was invisible and that his presence was transparent and meaningless.

The Second Dream: Six Months After the Beginning of Treatment

This dream occurred while we were discussing the emotional boundaries that Ami imposed on himself in our relationship and the question of what

1 At the time, children in Israeli Kibbutzim had to sleep away from their parents in the children's house and could see their parents only a few hours during the afternoon. Frequently this created difficulties for the parents.

would have happened if he had allowed himself more freedom to express his longing for me. These matters arose after the summer vacation, which was experienced as a frustrating interruption of our relationship.

The dream took place in the clinic. The atmosphere was relaxed but not routine:

> *I am observing the analysis of another patient, a friend from the past. I couldn't understand why the friend was in your clinic, which made me uneasy. Then the friend left and asked me to keep in touch with him. The discomfort continued. In fact, another woman was present in the room, perhaps a patient or student of yours. I felt unable to speak freely. There was a couch in the corner of the room, and you lay on it. The student said that you were not in a good state, and you nodded your head at me to confirm her words. Later, somebody else came in; it was probably your husband. He shook my hand and guessed my age. His estimate concluded that I was much older than I am, and I was surprised that your husband thought I was that old.*

In the associations, Ami expressed two simultaneous feelings. On the one hand, he could not speak to me freely due to the presence of the others. On the other hand, he was curious about those others but thought that there was a kind of forbidden voyeurism in this curiosity. I linked these associations to my having been away on vacation, the interruption to our being together, and Ami wondering who those people I was with were.

This talk allowed the patient to be more openly interested in the "others" who appeared in the dream. I suggested that they were parts of his self; for example, the friend from the past was his pre-traumatic self-representation, including his longing to preserve its wholesome essence. The girl was a representation of female elements in his self. I pointed out that each of these self-representations is disconnected from the others, and this disconnection, in and of itself, produces discontent. At the same time, the possibility of gathering all these self-representations in one room in my clinic suggests the beginning of a process of restoration. The therapist lying on the couch, I suggested, was a representation of his wounded self and a sense of affinity that emerged between her and him through simultaneous experiencing. That she, like him, is wounded perhaps suggests a sort of substitution in the Levinasian sense, wounded instead of him and now being in his state.

In continuing to work on this dream, Ami said that many of his current dreams were connected to his pre-injury self. He thought that he might in any case have been affected by feelings of basic insecurity, even if he had not been injured, because of the accumulation of empathic failures he had experienced within his environment. However, it seemed to him that the trauma of the injury seemed to have erased all pre-traumatic experiences because, in light of this colossal injury, all other events had lost meaning. The dream work we are now engaged in Ami's therapy enables him to establish a new potential space in which he can assemble all the different events which had previously plagued him. In this space, there is room for the pre-traumatic little boy as well as the presently wounded son. The fact is that since the injury, he felt that he was required to be "big" to deal with the disasters endured by "adults." He connected this subject to my partner's estimate of his age, which saw him as older than he actually was.

Later on, we realized that in this dream, the patient's dual use of the therapist is particularly interesting: She is lying lifeless on the couch and carrying the patient's illness and deadness. In her maternal preoccupation and as a selfobject, she cannot remain unaffected by the severe trauma of her analytic child and experiences the patient's agony. If the child is injured, the therapist is also injured. At the same time, the image of the therapist resonates with the memory of his mother, injured in the hammock, cut off from him and unreachable. In other words, the dream unfolds both the current situation and the memory from the past. Even though the image itself is identical in both cases, there is a major difference between the two. The analytic object is different from the archaic object; the therapist communicates with him with subtle signs that only he understands, resembling the private language of a mother and her baby, conveying that she sees him and that her attention is focused on him.

Hearing this interpretation, Ami spoke of missing and longing to be with me exclusively, continuously and without interruptions. He did not want to grow up prematurely within our shared work. This expressed his longing to relive what he had been previously deprived of – experiencing the secure tie of a child with his mother without interruptions.

Ami also expressed surprise at the appearance of my partner as a possible paternal figure, though he had no memory of his father, with the exception of those events and accidents that had led him to be hospitalized. This comment implied the possible expansion of the transitional space and the prospect of the inclusion of a father figure in the mother–child dyad.

The Third Dream: The Beginning of the Third Year

During this phase, Ami was preoccupied with pictures of his childhood and with feelings of anger toward his parents, who had always been mostly engaged in their own lives. This was especially true of his reserved mother and detached father. At this time, he experienced the relationship with me as dependable and felt that in this room, he could give himself enough freedom to emerge. He was determined to relinquish what he defined as his "emotional disability," which included breaking up with a girl who, he felt, reinforced his annoying experience of being disabled.

In this context, an intense erotic infatuation developed in the transference, with talk of various fantasies regarding what could possibly occur between us. I was amazed at his ability to speak so openly about his physical need for bodily intimacy with me:

> In the dream, *I see you sitting with your back leaning against the wall. We get physically close and almost touch each other. In my thoughts I worry that your husband will see or hear us. I begin to undress you and wonder how you can continue to be my therapist. However, at the same time, I see that you are signaling that everything will be fine. Suddenly, I look at your legs and am surprised to see how thin they are. Concerned, I wonder what had happened to those legs and why they are so thin. You respond that they are thin but strong. I relax, knowing that the legs are strong.*

In his associations, Ami related the obstacles standing in the way of realizing the closeness with me. He drew attention to the fact that this time the obstacle was not external but came from within. The thought about my husband was now a kind of signifier of an internalized experience of possible disruption, a potential rather than an actual interruption. Alongside the worry, there is a sense of legitimacy, a positive anticipation and curiosity in regard to touch. The Oedipal connotations of the dream are obvious.

Conceivably, the more important meaning of the dream is the transformation that is evident in the use of the space of my clinic, the place where our relation exists. From using it as a container for the evacuation of horrific experiences, the space of the clinic turned into a place where hindrances can be contained, and needs are met by a selfobject. The therapist is not used anymore as a bearer of illness and death. Rather, at this point, she functions in a way that nourishes the patient's vitality and supports his emerging needs. At the same time, anxiety still hovers; the legs are "too thin" and maybe too weak to offer sufficient support. The therapist understands the patient's concern and indicates that the legs are "thin but strong."

Later, I suggested that maybe "legs" had become a symbol that promotes the therapeutic process. With their help, Ami reactivates and revives his inner legs, his ability to move in the broadest sense of the word. When my legs are present there and work to assure his confidence, a transmuting internalization of the experience of stability can occur; the stability of my legs becomes the stability of his legs. My presence and my communication nurture his faith in his own powers and offers mirroring and validation to the feeling that he is entitled to firm legs, and that is what he has. The fragmented self is now directed toward restoration. The disintegration fades and gives way to integration.

The Fourth Dream: The End of the Third Year

This dream was termed the "umbilical cord dream." I understood that the dream reflected a transformation in the transference relationship. The therapist no longer appears concretely, now that her function as a selfobject is sufficiently internalized.

The dream was recounted at a moment in time when the patient developed a relationship with a new girlfriend, and this included enjoying the intimate contact with her. His new girlfriend showed considerable empathic competence and patience. She unwaveringly helped him deal with physical difficulties in their intimate relationship. In the transference, a significant change took place. From an intense involvement with me and fantasies about intimacy and sexuality, Ami now saw me as a consistently available figure and someone who could be relied on unconditionally. At this stage he was immersed in the new possibilities he was discovering for himself, the encounter with his own vitality and excitement from these innovations. He began to think about ending treatment. At the same time, this thought of a possible termination also raised concerns that, without treatment, he would regress to the initial states of disintegration.

In this context, he narrated the following dream:

I am standing on the edge of a cliff, a place I remember from my childhood. Facing me was a deep ravine. Standing next to me was a boy I knew at school. I suggested to the friend that we go down the cliff with the help of ropes. He refused because he was afraid and suggested that I go down myself and he would observe me from above. I was also afraid of descending, wondering if the nail I had pinned into the rock would hold the rope and whether the rope was long enough to reach the bottom. I started to go down, and the friend followed me. I felt a kind of surprise when I discovered that the ravine was much deeper than I initially thought. I hadn't realized that the path would be so long. Then I remembered the miracle of the jug of oil,[2] *as the rope seemed to get longer and longer and unexpectedly reached the bottom of the abyss. I finally got there and met a man who told me I was brave and resourceful. I confessed to having been scared.*

Ami said that he woke up with a positive feeling, sensing that he was no longer restless and preoccupied with fears of losing control, as was evident in his first dreams. In this dream, he was actually able to organize his environment properly and control the situation but still feel fearful as well. He felt that he was progressing, accepting responsibility for what was happening and trusting himself more and more. He was not drawn to skeptical voices like that of his friend in the dream. This time, he had something to lean on, an umbilical cord, and someone to trust.

Deciphering the various experiences of the self that are enfolded in this dream took many hours. On the one hand, a worrying and skeptical aspect appeared that tended to preserve the tendency to withdraw from new experiences. Ami remembered his parents, who refrained from encouraging him to dare and "go forward." On the other hand, there was another aspect that pushed him ahead despite the anxiety. Now he wondered: would it be right to marry his girlfriend? Will he ever be able to have children? Such thoughts were virtually implausible in the past. I understood that the transformations, at this stage, were experienced with both excitement and anxiety.

In our relation, too, there appeared concerns about the depth of our relationship, along with a feeling that as long as he is connected to the umbilical cord, he will dare to move forward. I understood that Ami was concerned that the cord that linked us would be cut prematurely, and the danger of

2 The miracle of the jug of oil is a Jewish legend related to the uprising of the Hasmoneans, in 165 BC. There was a jug of oil in the holy temple that should have had enough oil to burn a lamp for one day. Unexpectedly, the oil lasted for eight days. Therefore, Jewish people have a festival, Hanukkah, and light candles for eight days during this holiday.

falling still existed. I suggested that at this stage of our work, unlike in the past, the umbilical cord belonged to him and that he could take it anywhere. The image of the cord indicates a transmuting internalization of the selfobject function, an analytic mother who is different from the archaic mother in the sense that her presence provides him with competence, confidence, and faith. This dream became a significant step in our shared experience and marked the beginning of our separation.

Fifth Dream: The End of the Fifth Year

For many months before this dream, the patient had dealt a great deal with the issue of the end of our joint journey. In numerous dreams, he found himself walking down an unmarked path, finding the passage blocked or encountering other unexpected obstacles. Most of these obstacles appeared at the very end of the path when it seemed that he had completed the course. We realized that our work was coming to an end, and we recognized the various difficulties as a sign of separation anxiety and unwillingness to give up our shared voyage.

In the midst of all this, the patient decided to get married. The following dream was reported six months after his marriage when various fantasies arose regarding the expected separation between us:

> *We are sitting side by side on a small wall on the Mount of Olives*[3] *and seeing the Old City opposite us. You show me the spectacular view, including the Dome of the Rock glistening in the sun, and I express the beauty of the sight. I look in another direction; my gaze intersects with the direction of your observation. I show you a sight that resembles an abstract painting. The appearance of the painting is not as clear as the view you show me. You look happy and comment that the sight I am showing you is beautiful.*

In his associations with the dream, Ami remembered a certain place in East Jerusalem, where he used to sit with his girlfriends on a low wall, with his legs dangling by the side of the wall. The place was suitable for intimate conversations, he explained. I thought he was hinting at the conversations we had at the clinic. Ami validated this idea and noted that this time, he

3 A mountain ridge in West Jerusalem.

took us outside to a boundless expanse of the landscape, to a place with special points of light, the Dome of the Rock. In this place, *he* could show *me* something. On further thought he explained that he must have shown me a reflection of what I had shown him: he remembered the windows of the Intercontinental Hotel on the Mount of Olives, in which the view of the Old City was reflected. Thus, he concluded that I showed him the view of the Old City while he showed me the reflection of the same view in the windows.

I pointed out a deep affinity between his vision and mine; we see the same things, each in his own version. This will be the case when we part. He will remain with the images we saw together, but they will belong to him, adapted to his personal adaptation, an expression of his subjective experiences.

Unlike the dreams of the past, especially the dream about the creature that shed blood and my partner appearing as an interrupting factor, this dream flowed freely and gave space to the gaze of each of us without disturbance. The images of his mind are now formed without disruptions and take shape in an endless interconnectedness with his environment.

Thinking back, I realized that the patient located the dream in front of the Gate of Mercy in the Old City, and above the cemetery, as if asking for rebirth, as do the dead who expect to be resurrected with the coming of the Messiah. The dream reveals him sitting "securely" on the wall, supported by the inner legs created within the therapeutic process. At that point in time, he was no longer in need of my legs or worried about their thinness but rather relied on his strong inner legs, legs that could be leaned on, be trusted, and be seen in his dream, like a virtual self that came into being during the therapy. Now, he can "hold" what is lacking while experiencing fullness; he was dreaming of his pre-traumatic self, the man he was before the injury, with his post-analytic self.

Epilogue

Ami started a family and had children. His fatherhood was a highly significant experience, and his devotion to his children aroused great respect. After years, he fell ill with a disease that gradually spread throughout his body. He was admitted to a hospital and requested that we go back to our conversations, now on the phone. When things got worse, I offered to visit him in the hospital. I knew this would be our last meeting.

While we were still sitting in the visitor's area, he told me about various dreams that plagued him during his hospitalization: large and small containers appeared again and again in his dreams. He explained that they were related to our relationship and my presence ingrained in his mind. I understood that Ami was telling me that he is sustained through an internalized selfobject function, knowing at this time that such a presence is necessary to preserve his vitality. Ami internalized the idea that his existence depends on the presence of those who are there for him, see him, hold him, and even inspire him.

This man, wounded by those who were supposed to protect him, could have collapsed into endless rage and bitterness, but instead, he achieved an admirable transformation and was able to believe in life and in those who have faith in holding on to it.

Shortly after our meeting, I received a message that Ami had passed away.

I visited the family during the seven-day period of mourning. His wife asked me to tell her and his children about Ami. I talked with them about his special personality, about his courage, about the integrity that characterized him, about his determination to live, to have children, and to realize the ideals that guided his life. I told them that despite his death, these ideals would continue to exist with them, inside their souls. I tried to talk to them about the infinity of these ideals and the possibility that those ideals would be like oxygen to their souls.

These ideals continued and continue to exist within me as well. He was one of the dearest people I ever knew.

May his memory be blessed.

The Wisdom of the Dream Work and the Area of Faith

The study of dreams has fascinated humans since ancient times. People used to travel to a holy place to receive a sign from God, a priest, or another heavenly being. In ancient Greece, the seeker of the answer used to go to a sacred place and expected to "receive" a special dream that would grant him wisdom and clarity of mind and sustain him. This line of thought considered that the dream may be a certain premonition or a prediction. One can speculate that the Greek Oracle was in fact the precursor of our contemporary analytic interpretation.

Nowadays, psychoanalytic thinking on dreams involves a range too broad to be fully described in this chapter. Therefore, I will offer only a few comments that place this dream work in a theoretical context. The origin of thinking about dreams is, of course, Freud's extensive work on the "Interpretation of Dreams," first published in 1900–01. Freud proposed to see the overt material of the dream as a camouflage for repressed latent materials, which are associated with psychic conflicts. Freud believed that by means of free associations, it is possible to decipher the hidden meaning of the dream's contents, the distortions of reality, as well as transferential aspects. These thoughts assume that the interpretation of the dream allows a restoration, even if partial, of the horizontal split.

Freud thought that traumatic dreams deserve special attention. He suggested that these dreams should be identified as a unique group in the sense that they stem from a compulsive need to re-experience traumatic situations, including an attempt to find a way to cope with the situation in a better manner. Hence, the dream does not only express a wish but is also used to find a solution to a traumatic situation.

Bion's (1977, pp. 65–85) chapter on hallucination expands Freud's thinking and proposes to investigate the dream work, which occurs not only at night but also during daytime waking hours. Such an investigation creates a continuum in mental life between waking (which is guided by fantasies) and sleep (which is guided by dreaming). Like hallucinations, daydreaming is a constant process. It expands the range of awareness and transforms the conscious mind into the unconscious by revealing the unconscious elements that are contained in conscious materials. This flexibility of the mind enables the analyst to detect significant changes in the patient's psyche and in the transference. There is a continual changeability between the conscious and the unconscious. In fact, we dream or daydream, even within the analytic hour. The patient relates his dream, and the therapist dreams it. This activity, much like myths,[4] promotes the transformation of the mind.

Winnicott (1965, 1971) referred to dreams as a zone of illusion, with special emphasis on the creativity inherent in it. He (1965, pp. 29–36)

4 In Bion's thinking myths are perceived as a kind of dreaming that has social meaning. The myth, like the dream, is based on overt material which requires deciphering and an understanding of concealing meaning. Dreams and myths express the remnants of daily experiences and ambiguous encounters. In the chapters of this book, there are references to various myths: Oedipus (Chapters 1 and 10), the Tower of Babel, the expulsion from the Garden of Eden, the story of the king of Thebes (Chapter 1), the Greek myth of Pygmalion and the Indian myth about Queen Simantini (Chapter 8), and the myth of Odysseus (Chapter 11). All these serve the thought processes of the alpha function, and deciphering them contributes to the expansion of the mind.

suggested that the dream fulfills a holding function, works for time–space cohesion, and sustains one singular self that contains all elements. It seeks to consolidate the integration of the dissociated or split experiences of the self. This function of the dream instigates the development of a creative transitional space and is always dependent on the presence of another.

Winnicott's followers also proposed that man's creative capacity, his ability to indulge in playfulness, always depends on a certain context (Bollas, 1987, 1989, 1992). Hence, we can assume that the ability to dream and to interpret the dream creatively is contingent on the presence of the analyst, since the dream is brought to a certain analyst at a certain stage of the treatment.

Kohut, in dialogue with classical psychoanalysis, presented a different approach to dreams. Unlike Freud, who saw the visible material as a marker for deeper unconscious meanings that require deciphering, Kohut (1971) suggested that the overt material is fascinating in itself. Many dreams reflect the psychological self-state of the dreamer. The dream work allows the dissolving of the vertical split alongside the dismantling of the horizontal split.

Kohut distinguished between two types of dreams: a patient who is not on the verge of a breakdown comes with dreams that deal with love, jealousy, and various conflicts. They do not threaten his well-being. We use his associations to merge into his inner world. Unlike these patients, who are mainly neurotic, in patients with narcissistic injuries, or those who are on the verge of disintegration, the content of the dream indicates falling walls and experiences of disintegration. Our interpretation of these situations strives for the restoration of horror and the construction of flexible walls (Mann, 2014). Here, the central issues of the self are manifested in an undisguised manner, and it is obvious that the drive overwhelms the fragmented self. Dream work with these patients mainly requires a validating presence. It is important that the therapist acknowledges the horror and a kind of chronic helplessness.

The first dream is an example of this type of horror dream, where fragmentation, perversion and helplessness dominate the subjective experience.

Kohut also suggests taking an interest in dreams as structuring the patients' childhood experiences that arise within the analysis and relating them to the analyst within any given hour (Strozier, 2001). He recommends that the interpretation of dreams would always come after listening to the patient's words and his associations, and only when the therapist felt that he understood the dream sufficiently would he offer an interpretation.

Beyond relating to the different theories on dreaming, my work was focused on weaving an area of faith that greatly contributed to the restoration of the patient's painful wounds. Eigen (1981) formulated the concept of the "area of faith" and defined it as "prostration with all the heart, all the soul and all possible" (p. 413). The formation of the area of faith illuminates an important function of the selfobject; it consists of a moment of mutual exploration and joint creativity of the therapist and the patient. Each one is an active agent as well as a passive recipient of thoughts, and within this fabric, new meanings and potentialities evolve.

In Ami's dreams, one can find that the analyst provides an anticipatory echo (Kulka, 2005),[5] a "voice" that intuits that the situation is safe and not disintegrating. This is a leap to nonlinear quantum thinking, obscure at times and clear at other moments, which is based on the area of faith. In the first dream, the therapist cleans the table; in the second dream, the injured therapist nods in the patient's direction and gives a sign of calmness; in the third dream, she signals to him that "everything is fine" despite the erotic infatuation which involves danger. In the fourth dream about the umbilical cord, there is evidence of the selfobject function that establishes confidence. In the final dream, there is a jump into a supra-individual transitional space of mirrors and reflections.

Trauma usually works to restrict the area of faith. The wounded self produces elaborate strategies and defense mechanisms that block the natural emergence of the potentiality of the self. In its wounded state, the self is fragmented, frozen, distorted, and rigid. Is this a permanent situation or is the fragmented state impermanent and changeable? Our work demonstrates the possibility of cultivating compensatory mechanisms that contribute to the restoration of the self, its vitality, and its lost potential (Kohut, 2009).[6]

5 In the introduction to the Hebrew translation of Kohut's *How Does Analysis Cure?*, Kulka (2005) suggests the concept of "anticipatory echo." He explains that an anticipatory echo does not describe what exists but is rather "a harbinger of the self's existence. Selfhood is always contingent on the anticipatory echo that precedes it. The completeness of the self is based on this paradox."

6 Kohut (2009) distinguishes between defense mechanisms and compensatory structures. A compensatory structure resembles the original structure, except that the original structure did not develop from the start. The analysis attempts to construct compensatory structures instead of defense mechanisms. The defense mechanism has the quality of survival; it holds the self so that it does not collapse and is possessed by an intensity that cannot always be transformed. At times, perversion exemplifies these situations.

However, if there are still "remnants" in the psyche of good a nurturing experience, they can be the "seeds" from which it may be possible to cultivate a compensatory structure. The possibility of creating compensatory structures instead of defense mechanisms occurs via an adapted, empathetic presence, an active acceptance of the patient, and lending the therapist's mind to a collective mental effort.

"Thin but Strong legs" is an example of the formation of a compensatory structure. The umbilical cord dream is an example of the symbolized ideal selfobject, which fosters an experience of safety, reliable presence and security. It is a compensatory structure as well. Castrating and disrupted experiences transform into a continuous experience of hope and faith. There is an evolution in the transference, which has occurred due to the steadiness of the analytical process.

A Last Thought: Dreaming and Meditation

At the end of this chapter, I would like to offer another thought regarding dreaming alongside the other psychoanalytic meanings. We assume that the dream illuminates the dark areas, the hidden or neglected ones of the psyche, and turns them into significant elements in the mind. The visual imagery suggests connotations that are not usually easily deciphered; it is not based on learned knowledge, nor on conceptual language, but on an intuitive understanding of the subjective experiences in preverbal terms.

In this sense, dreaming is similar to meditative states. It consists of a search for profound meaning and strives to purify the soul from its toxic experiences. Meditation is designed to face the inner reality, to make peace with it, to transform haunting and painful inner experiences through intuiting new possibilities, different versions than those that usually guide the self. The meditator is in a spiritual state of mind and explores repetitive attachments that cause suffering.[7] He adjusts himself to certain states of mind, just as the dreamer puts a spotlight on his dreams on the images of the internal theater of the mind. The meditator works to concentrate on the object of the meditation just as the dreamer focuses his awareness on a certain dream object. This is how a bridge was built, in both cases, between the deceptive immediate reality, which contracts the mind, and the recognition of a broad ultimate reality, which promotes an expansion of the mind.

Various meditations are actually based on a type of daydreaming. For example, in meditating on mental clarity, we begin by focusing the concentration on the breath, then, we choose a mental "picture," an object of meditation. For instance, we imagine lying on a mountain peak and looking at the clear, cloudless sky. We visualize an empty space, much like that

7 See Chapter 11 on emptiness and equanimity as methods for evacuating the mind from thoughts that create suffering.

sky. From time to time, we encounter thoughts that divert our attention but treat them as passing clouds. Clarity of mind is attained by focusing on one continuous meditation object.

Tonglen is another, more complex meditation, which means "give and take" (McDonald, 2005). The purpose of this practice is to cultivate compassion. This requires the visualization of projecting clean and pure air into the world and inhaling black toxic air, that is, introjecting the suffering around us. Other meditations involve the visualization of figures of different Buddhas with different attributes and a guided visualization of the white and black smoke.

There is no doubt that dreaming and meditating are not identical. At the same time, both practices consist of imagery, whether it is dreaming or intentional visualization. These dreamy or imagined images are metaphors for the unknown and facilitators for possible associations to a dream or as insights in meditation. That is, images are a medium for investigating states of the mind and expanding it. Ami's dream work is an example of this mental effort to purify the mind from its poisonous contents.

References

Bion, W. R. (1977). *Second thoughts: Selected papers on psycho-Analysis*. J. Aronson.

Bollas, C. (1987). *The shadow of the object: Psychoanalysis of the unthought known*. Columbia University Press.

Bollas, C. (1989). *Forces of destiny: Psychoanalysis and human idiom*. Free Association Books.

Bollas, C. (1992). *Being a character: Psychoanalysis and self experience*. Hill and Wang.

Eigen, M. (1981). The area of faith in Winnicott, Lacan and Bion. *The International Journal of Psycho-Analysis*, *62*(4), 413–433.

Freud, S. (1953). The interpretation of dreams. In J. Strachley & A. Freud (Eds.), *The standard edition of the complete psychological works of Sigmund Freud: Vols. 4 & 5 (1900–1901): The interpretation of dreams (First and Second Parts)*. Hogarth Press.

Kohut, H. (1971). *The analysis of the self: A systematic approach to the psychoanalytic treatment of narcissistic personality disorders*. International Universities Press.

Kohut, H. (2009). *The restoration of the self*. The University of Chicago Press.

Kulka, R. (2005). Between tragedy and compassion (in Hebrew). In H. Kohut (Ed.), *How does analysis cure?* (E. Idan, Trans., Hebrew ed., pp. 13–52). Am Oved Publishers.

Mann, G. (1998). From disintegration to unintegration: The creation of potential space through work with dreams. *Journal of the American Academy of Psychoanalysis, 26*(3), 389–416. https://doi.org/10.1521/jaap.1.1998.26.3.389
Mann, G. (2014). Flexible walls: The analytic frame as the creative context. *Ma'arag: The Israel Annual of Psychoanalysis, 5*, 153–169.
McDonald, K. (2005). *How to meditate: A practical guide* (R. Courtin, Ed.). Wisdom Publications.
Strozier, C. B. (2001). *Heinz Kohut: The making of a psychoanalyst*. Farrar, Straus and Giroux.
Winnicott, D. W. (1965). *The maturational processes and the facilitating environment: Studies in the theory of emotional development*. Hogarth Press.
Winnicott, D. W. (1971). *Playing and reality*. Basic Books.

Chapter 10

Emptiness, Equanimity, and the Selfobject Function

Introduction

The main characteristic of our being self psychologists is our profound conviction that the presence of one person constitutes the selfhood of another. This profound contextual perspective was first introduced by Kohut and later adopted as a basic assumption in the community of self psychology. We believe that obtaining understanding is the first step in a good self psychology therapy and that this can be attained via empathy and by fulfilling a selfobject function for our patients.

This connectedness with our patients is not just an ordinary verbal interaction. In fact, it is our transformative presence that evokes and brings out in the patient what is disavowed, disguised, or unrealized. We assume an infinite openness to changeability and provide nonintrusive support.[1] We do not stick to one interpretation, nor are we the analysts who "know it all." We are endlessly attuned to and immersed in the micro-changes of the selfobject matrix, which constitutes the patient's state of mind. Such presence cultivates possible transformations of the mind.

In his seminal paper, "Forms and Transformations of Narcissism," Kohut (1966) coined the concept of "selfobject function." He concerned himself with the transformations of narcissism and believed that the selfobject presence supports the modification of archaic narcissism into a more mature narcissism. In the paper, Kohut claims that when the cohesive self is secure enough to relinquish its personal narcissistic goals, it can dissolve into a new psychological configuration far removed from any previous personality structure. It can transcend to an "expanded self which includes the world" (Kohut, 1966, p. 260). Such development is possible via five

1 Unknown support, a concept that Eigen (1998) used.

DOI: 10.4324/9781003449386-10

transformations of narcissism that he delineated: creativity, empathy, accepting transience, humor, and wisdom. These transformations constitute what Kohut defined as "cosmic narcissism." They reflect alterations in narcissism that have substantial transcendental value.

Yet Kohut never specified how we can bring about these transformations (Lachmann, 2007). Lachmann only cautiously remarked that "there is only a limited possibility for an expansion of the human capacity in these directions" (2007, p. 72). Even when asked directly about these transformations in one of the Chicago lectures, Kohut (1996) could not provide a clear response that would indicate how such modifications occur. He presented clinical material to illustrate the enormous significance of a well-balanced narcissistic matrix. The implied answer was that transformations occur in the presence of idealized selfobjects.

We assume that it is relatively easy to demonstrate the nature of creativity and humor. They are visible in the clinical encounter and appear in psychoanalytic literature from its earliest days. Empathy too appears in multiple psychoanalytic narratives, but it is not usually depicted in the distinctive manner in which Kohut elaborated it, namely that observer and the observed are inseparable. For Kohut (1982), empathy or vicarious introspection makes up the analyst's capacity to enter another person's mind to experience the world approximately from that person's perspective, "to put oneself in the other person's shoes." It is certainly not easy to achieve the high level that Kohut required for true empathy. It is apparently even more difficult to comprehend and demonstrate the ideas of wisdom and the acceptance of transience. It may be that the metaphysical nature or complexity of these transformations makes them difficult to illustrate. Since we wish to comprehend the transformations to wisdom and transience more clearly, we ask whether we can enrich ourselves through knowledge of Buddhist concepts and practice methods. The Buddhist tradition offers practice methods that enhance wisdom and promote the acceptance of impermanence. Such practice consists of close observation of the mind; the mind's emotional logic, its lucid moments as well as its false representations. It is important to recall that Buddhist philosophy was intended to deal with and cure human suffering.

The Bodhisattva as a Selfobject

One Buddhist idea that comes to mind when thinking about transformations of narcissism is that of the Bodhisattva (Mann, 2013, 2015). Most people live by their desires and ambitions to attempt to gain material advantage. In distinction, according to Buddhist tradition, there is the Bodhisattva, an ordinary person who attained Nirvana because of being enlightened and released from suffering, who takes up a different course in his or her life. The Bodhisattva adopts the vow to help all sentient living beings and to protect the helpless and the needy. This vow is not an emotional stance but an ethical promise that is meant to prevail irrespective of whether another person is a close friend or a stranger. This humane position consists of a profound faith in human nature.

The concept of the Bodhisattva reminds us of Kohut's (1984) concepts of "being human among humans" (p. 200) and fulfilling a selfobject function. It is possible to think of the selfobject function as a self psychology version of the Bodhisattva function. Both strive to realize the idea of transforming personal narcissism to a higher form of narcissism, what Kohut refers to as supra-individual existence in the world. As mentioned earlier, this state of selfhood was defined by him as cosmic narcissism. It diminishes duality, not in the Freudian sense of a "one person psychology" but as a transcendental experience that cultivates an extension of personal subjectivity.

In Buddhist tradition, it is believed that anyone may be a Bodhisattva since all people have a Buddha nature within themselves. Yet it is not enough just to be familiar with the idea of a Bodhisattva. It is more important to accept the actions of a Bodhisattva and to cultivate them as a direct experience within one's own mind.

A metaphor for such cultivation of the mind is the idea that the mind is a storage of infinite varieties of seeds: seeds of suffering, seeds of enlightenment, seeds of greed and seeds of generosity, and seeds of sorrow and seeds of happiness (Hanh, 2001). These negative and positive seeds may propel us to bad or good directions. Cultivating the mind implies assuming the task of a gardener who waters those seeds that give rise to wisdom and compassion and help them grow. With such mindfulness, our thinking and actions gravitate in the direction of healing and transformation. Ghent (2001) also uses the metaphor of gardening in his discussion of techniques for cultivating new needs as opposed to elaborating repetitive patterns. His ideas were also inspired by Buddhist thinking. He argues that needs may be created in certain circumstances:

> A question that frequently arises (or should arise) in the course of psychoanalysis is whether, at any moment, to water the flowers or to locate and pull out the weeds – whether to focus on what is new and different

> (non-transference) in the realm of perception, need, and action or to focus on what is old and, in important respects, repetitive (transference). The latter can be seen not only as transference but also as resistance to something new that is trying to emerge.
>
> (Ghent, 2001, p. 34)

In fact, cultivating the mind consists of continuous exploration of the potential evolution of the primordial still-not-traumatized self and the link to Buddha nature. With an attuned selfobject position, we are striving to eliminate vertical splits and enhance interconnectedness within human experiences (Mann, 2013).

Transformations of the Mind: The Selfobject Function, Emptiness, and Equanimity

As we look in more detail at Buddhist teachings, we come to identify various references to possible transformations of the mind. Mahayana Buddhism defines six "Paramitas," namely six stages of perfection of the mind or realization of certain virtues. The six virtues are generosity, morality, patience, diligence, meditation, and, the last and most important, wisdom. These virtues are cultivated as a way of refinement and purification of karma. Practice is aimed at helping the aspirant live an unobstructed life while reaching the goal of enlightenment.

Wisdom is the ultimate virtue that includes all other virtues. If generosity is the initial realization of the dharma, then wisdom is its definitive realization and is implied in the other Paramitas in alternate forms. Through the practice of the other virtues – generosity, morality, patience, diligence, and meditation – a person cultivates wisdom.

The concept of wisdom is based on the insightful understanding that all phenomena lack self-essence, that is, they are empty of inherent existence.[2] Therefore, it is assumed that the realization of emptiness and its correlate, equanimity, promote and constitute wisdom. How do the concepts of emptiness and equanimity[3] contribute to the promotion of wisdom? How does wisdom connect to the idea of being a selfobject?

2 See the discussion on transience in Chapter 7.

3 Equanimity (known as *upekkha*) is a spiritual virtue that means accepting gain and loss, good-repute and ill-repute, praise and censure, sorrow, and happiness, all with detachment,

Emptiness makes it possible not to use our wisdom just to enhance our own state of well-being for the sake of our own enlightenment but to offer our wisdom to our fellow human beings so as to promote their well-being to support enlightenment for others. This attitude is considered to be the highest transformative state of the mind. It is the attitude that characterizes the Bodhisattwa as well as the selfobject. In other words, to be a true selfobject or, in Buddhist terms, be a Bodhisattva, one needs to realize emptiness. Such a realization constitutes wisdom.

We realize that emptiness is a complex concept. It is founded on the realization that no phenomenon has an inherent existence. Infinite transformation, impermanence, is a trait of all phenomena. Attachment to any particular preference, perspective, or understanding is bound to create hindrances to the promotion of wisdom. The practice of relieving suffering requires that one empties oneself from preconceptions and personal desires so as to be receptive to living in the moment as it comes, accepting the moment with no attachment to prior ideas. A well-known image for such a state of mind is the idea of "mirror consciousness."[4] Like the mirror, our mind does not attach itself to anything and does not refuse anything. This is what is called "emptiness."

Bion (1984b, 1988), who was also informed by Eastern philosophy, defined this situation clearly in his highly regarded idea that the analyst works without memory, without desire, and without understanding.[5] He put em-

---

equally for oneself and for others. It is a tranquil state of mind, not succumbing to delusions, mental distress, or agitation. Equanimity is the last of four mental positions that are defined in the Brahma Virhas. They are also known as the four immeasurables. They include loving kindness, compassion, empathic joy, and equanimity.

4 "The perfect man uses his mind like a mirror – going after nothing, welcoming nothing, responding but not storing" (Chuang Tzu, 1968, p. 97).

5 Compare to Suzuki (1970) on emptiness:

> When you study Buddhism you should have a general house cleaning of your mind. You must take everything out of your room and clean thoroughly. If it is necessary, you may bring everything back in again. But if they are not necessary, there is no need to keep them.
>
> (pp. 111–112)

Compare also to Freud (1958):

> As soon as anyone deliberately concentrates his attention to a certain degree, he begins to select from the material before him. This however, is precisely what must not be done. In making this selection . . . he is in danger of never finding anything but what he already knows.
>
> (pp. 111–112)

phasis on the importance of a process of intuitive receptivity to an unknown truth to enable a transformation in O, "at-one-ment" with a non-articulate ultimate reality. Such a transformation is expressed in the capacity to reconnect to the vast chain of human events, subdued to a transcendental position (Grotstein, 2000).[6] The human mind may then transcend its personal dimension to a transpersonal existence, an ultimate existence.

From this point of view, the inspiration is to connect with ideas that are not thought yet or those that are not yet appropriated by a thinker (Bion, 1984a) to comprehend something that is beyond the immediate perception. This is not a theological idea in which the transcendental transformation is derived from an external source, God, but consists of the immanent transcendence of the human mind based on its capacity to transcend its personal dimensions to an ultimate experience (Mann, 2007). Bion, similarly to Kohut, introduced the idea but did not explain to us how to train ourselves to attain the "not-knowing," "empty" state of mind. And what does it really mean for the analyst to be "empty"? Is it the neutrality and abstinence that Freud (1958) recommended? In fact, we know that Freud failed to be abstinent or "empty" when it came to his beloved patients.

So what are emptiness and the state of "not-knowing"? The main point that I wish to emphasize is that emptiness is a state of mind of the analyst when she applies herself as a selfobject. Being a selfobject – immersed in empathy, not in identification – is similar to what Buddhists define as "emptiness." In this state, the selfobject renounces his or her personal narcissistic needs.

Buddhist wisdom teaches us how to train the mind to preserve a state of emptiness so as to be able to welcome any "guest" with mindfulness, whether there is a preconceived positive thought or a threatening negative one. With emptiness and its correlation, equanimity, it is possible to relate to all experiences as equally significant and deserve our total compassion.

Let us take the simple example of water. Water is a source of life for the thirst; it is a habitat of living for fish; it is a prerequisite for the growth of trees and plants; it is a source of energy; it may appear as a wave, whereas a moment later, it may be totally flat, part of the sea. Water does not have any one particular function or appearance. The function is determined by the

6 See especially the chapter "Why Oedipus and not Christ? (pp. 219–253).

specific context. Like other phenomena, water has different functions and different manifestations in different contexts; it is empty of one formative connotation.[7]

Thich Nhat Hanh (2001), a Vietnamese Buddhist monk and eminent teacher of Buddhism, distinguishes between different dimensions of reality: a conventional reality and an ultimate reality. We may consider that what we see is conventional reality; we comprehend the world as we sense it and know it. We realize that things are labeled and have accepted designations. Such conventional truth includes what is perceived, people we personally like or dislike, and the daily occurrences around us. This includes understandings of the world as it functions, as it manifests itself in our perceptions. However, there is also the ultimate dimension. It transcends the split way in which we ordinarily perceive the world, as Hanh (2001) describes:

> As long as we are caught in (conventional) notions. . ., we cannot arrive at true understanding, and we will not reach the ultimate dimension. . . . Insight is only possible when we see through notions of inside and outside, self and other. We realize that concepts such as one and many, coming and going, collective and individual, above and below, cannot be applied to ultimate reality.
>
> (p. 78)

This is the apperception of an ultimate dimension, the O, in Bion's terms. Here, there is no dualism. It is important to emphasize that emptiness here does not refer to nothingness or nihilism. It refers to the fact that, ultimately, our day-to-day experience of reality can be "empty" of many qualities that we normally assign to it since it is infinitely changing.

Hanh shows his students a cup of tea and asks: What is in the cup? The immediate answer, of course, is tea. And where did the tea come from? From the thermos. And where does the water in the thermos come from? From the river. In other words, when we look at the cup of tea, we see the

7 "Please Call Me by My True Names," a poem written in 1978 by Thich Nhat Hanh (2022, pp. 92–94), presents a useful exposition of the notion of emptiness. In this powerful poem, Hanh introduces the idea that nothing has a permanent essence. The self can be a frog swimming happily in a pond, and it can be the snake who feeds on the frog; it can be a young girl, raped by a pirate, and it can be the pirate who raped the girl. All phenomena have nothing but a contextual transitory appearance.

thermos, the river, the rain, and the rain clouds. This illustrates the ultimate dimension, as opposed to merely seeing the thermos and the tea. Things do not come into existence or cease to be but reveal themselves under certain circumstances and lose the quality of presence when circumstances change. That which is invisible is not nonexistent; it may exist as a seed in the reservoir of our awareness, a seed that can be watered or dried out. Emptiness means not being drawn into any particular manifestation.

The self, too, has similar dimensions. It is not an isolate; neither is it a fixed entity. We need to conceive of the idea that the self – in different circumstances – presents in different manifestations. All these manifestations are part of one potential self. We must especially take note of the fact that the wounded self may be dissociated, split, fragmented, or disintegrated. It may be totally invisible at one point and emerge fully at another point in time and circumstance. So if we search for a deep conviction of "what is the real self?", we come to the conclusion that there is no "independent self"; the self, too, lacks a steady and independent substance. There is an impermanent self, a self that has infinite cohesive manifestations into which its vast potential can be actualized. Infinite potentiality is the underlying bedrock of all possible states.

We accept infinite oscillations between potentiality and formation, dissolving and emergence (Kulka, 1997, 2012; Sucharov, 1992). We renounce our conventional concepts about the self's health or pathology and posit the assumption that emotional problems are transient, everlasting fluctuations of the self. We cultivate the belief that a suitable selfobject matrix promotes healing and reduces suffering. The self cannot possibly be independent or self-sufficient; it needs suitable circumstances for the realization of its ultimate quality at any moment. The context of a suitable selfobject matrix encourages the emergence of the primordial – untraumatized selfhood. Sometimes, the empty quality of the self is referred to as "no self."[8] This designation emphasizes the idea of no singularity, of emptiness. It is important to call attention to the idea that "emptiness" or "no self" is not selflessness, nor is it the annihilation of the self. With mindfulness, one can relinquish one's perception of a particular "I," physically as well as men-

8 A saying about the "no self" is Master Dōgen's famous claim:

> To study and learn the way of the Buddha, is to study and learn your own self. To study and learn your own self is to forget yourself. To forget is to be realized by the myriad things of the universe.
>
> (Dōgen, 1994, p. 370)

tally. We allow for the emergence of new perspectives in regard to ourselves and the "other."[9] We touch on the pre-reflexive self, still unconditioned by conventional dimensions.

To put it differently, renouncing one's own self is the precondition to immersing freely with the other's self, getting into her or his shoes and possibly sharing their experiences. When we accept the profound concept of interbeing and interconnectedness, including the never-ending changeability that is promoted by coexisting entities, we also comprehend that being attached to a particular idea about how the self must be or into which direction it should develop restricts the inner freedom that we wish to grant to our patients' selves.

Vignette I: Emptiness

A patient tells me that she came to the session after a great deal of preparation. At the beginning of the session, she announced that she wanted to talk to me about her frustration and anger with me. She felt that this ability to express discontent is something that she has gained in the course of our work of seven years in analysis. She felt entitled to express it out loud. She went on to tell me how lonely and helpless she feels because "she knows" that I am unable to share the suffering she experiences as a single woman. She knows (even though I never discussed it with her) that I married relatively early in my life, and she assumes that I cannot possibly comprehend the misery of a single woman. She believed that because I was never in such a situation, I lacked the ability to be with her in this regard. She explained that what she was saying was presented to me deliberately and in a "contained" manner; it was not, she wanted to say, an impulsive, angry outburst. She said that she was devastated by this missing link in my empathic capability.

Even though we discussed this issue many times before, the way she presented her feelings on that particular day threw me instantly, this time, into

9 The example refers to the need to avoid becoming attached to the teachings of Dharma (Buddhist wisdom). One may use the teachings and then let go of them. Here, we may refer to the metaphor of "The Raft" (Alagaddupama Sutra), which is given in the context of a discussion of the need of renunciation for the sake of emptiness. One needs a raft to cross the river, but once we have crossed the river, one can leave the raft behind. Holding on to the raft, after having crossed the river, signifies rigidity, attachment to fixed ideas, to known patterns, blindness, and therefore a hindrance to reach new solutions.

the mental state of a helpless woman in her forties who is unable to manage the task of finding sufficient love in her life and cannot constitute a family. I felt that I was suddenly thrown into this devastating situation. I imagined all the things that I would be deprived of, those which could have happened yet did not. I clearly had the sensation of an incomplete life at that moment. . . . Then, my mind sprang to thoughts about my motherhood: what kind of a mother am I, who cannot furnish my analytic daughter with enough feminine stock to go about life and find her own happiness? A cloud of deep sadness overcame me. I realized that I was probably experiencing some aspect of the dissatisfying and insufficient motherhood that she had been immersed in for so many years. I felt how tragic and disastrous this was for *her and for me*, for both of us as "daughter" and as "mother" interchangeably. Along with my grief, I also respected the fact that she did not want to be with such a mother anymore.

I told her that I may have denied her something that she should have gotten from me: the motherly inspiration that every daughter is entitled to get from her mother and that I was apparently unable to give to her. I could not be there in the way she needed me. "My hand was too short" (a Hebrew expression). This is a very difficult situation for her. I told her that it may be that I am not suited to help her in this particular respect. I had tears in my eyes. I could not hide my pain and did not want to.

The next day, she came in and shared a dream:

> I had a special dream; it is related to you. I thank God that I woke up by chance; otherwise, I would not have recalled the dream. *It is strange. There was an event on the lower floor of your house. It was related to the end of the year and there were about ten to twenty girls, each connected to you somehow. I was aware that I am connected to you therapeutically. I realized that you have other "favorites" but I did not mind that too much. There was a ceremonial atmosphere and perhaps someone read something. Perhaps a movie was shown.*

Here is the main point:

> *There was a child, perhaps aged three-four or seven-eight, who was very sweet. The boy said something that was amazing; none of us could have said such a thing. It was a complex and wise sentence: "When I am sad, I am happy, and then I can be sad." It seems to be a childish*

> *contradiction, but it was not. It was a profound idea. There were three steps: sadness, happiness, and sadness. Even now, I can hardly repeat it.*

In her free associations about this dream, she said that it was very natural that I would have a small boy. She thought that it was clear that she was the boy, as well as one of the girls. She continued:

> *It is connected to something that you said about sadness, and I could be happy about that. Maybe it means that where one can be immersed in sadness, in the presence of the other, one can also be truly happy. I feel significant when you sense my sadness.*

Transforming the self via the function of being a selfobject is enhanced through adherence to the principles of emptiness and impermanence. In the example, the patient was able to renounce her sadness when she felt that I experienced her pain not as part of the transference or countertransference but as a fellow human being, a daughter, a mother, a woman. It is the shared human experience which is not reducible to a specific interpretation. This enables her to feel happiness. Sadness and happiness are interchangeable emotions that come and go in the mind. This paradoxical and seemingly contradictory truth needs to be cultivated in the mind of the analyst before it can be conveyed to the minds of our patients.

We can appreciate Suzuki's (1970) formulation:

> By wisdom we do not mean some particular faculty or philosophy (or interpretation). It is the readiness of the mind that is wisdom. So wisdom could be various philosophies and teachings, and various kinds of research and studies. . . . Wisdom is not something to learn. Wisdom is something that comes out of your mindfulness. So the point is to be ready for observing things, and to be ready for thinking. This is called emptiness of your mind.
>
> (p. 15)

Equanimity

Equanimity, as mentioned earlier, is the foundation that permits emptiness and supports it profoundly. When our state of mind is equanimous, we can listen to anything that patients or others tell us in an open and accepting manner, and we do not give way to emotional upheavals. With such equanimity, it is possible to relate to different thoughts and people as equally important and renounce conventional assumptions. One can meet emptiness. We know that Kohut recommended that we cultivate infinite empathy, even toward those who committed crimes against humanity.

The profound significance of equanimity is the possibility of attending to different states of mind in a contemplative manner without collapsing into a splitting-conflictual mode.[10] Each form, or each manifestation, is accepted in its suchness as they are; they are not perceived as a contradiction to another situation.[11] We acknowledge existential circumstances without judgment.

A possible analogy can be drawn between the Buddhist concept of equanimity and the Indian Hindu concept of "rasa" (essence, juice, or taste in Sanskrit). Rasa connotes an essential, intrinsic emotional state that is created by the state of mind and is artistically presented. It may well be a primary feeling that is evoked in the actor as well as in the viewer. Despite the significant difference between equanimity and rasa, the Hindu scholar Abhinavagupta suggests that achieving a rasa experience requires a process of "universalization". In this process, individuals set aside their personal feelings and connect with a pure essence of emotions such as love, fear or peacefulness. The standard example refers to the spectator's seeing a fictive lion on the stage; one feels fear, not as fear for one's safety – since the spectator knows that the lion is a fiction – but rather a sort of abstracted fear. It is a stable and abstract connection not dependent on the individual context or the individual experience.[12] Therefore, rasa may be useful as a means to appreciate the meaning of

10 Buddhism offers practices to cultivate equanimity. First, we concentrate on situations that evoke pleasant compassionate feelings, situations in which it is easy to experience empathy. Once this is accomplished, we try to maintain such feelings toward increasingly difficult subjects, including those with whom we are less familiar and subjects toward whom we have grievances, anger, or even rage. We try to preserve our receptivity and to keep our openness to any subject or any topic that comes into mind.

11 The famous saying is, "When you sit, you sit. When you eat, you eat" (Suzuki, 1970, p. 42). He develops Master Dōgen's idea that form is form, and emptiness is emptiness. We can be in situations, whether they are good or bad, without disturbance or without being annoyed by feeling.

12 Prof. David Shulman, personal communication.

equanimity in one important sense: rasa is apprehended as an impersonal contemplative mood in its suchness without submitting to it or responding to it.

The wisdom of this extraordinary art lies in the dissolution of personal reactions and the adoption of an impersonal equanimous attitude, which is believed to be its highest mode of being. It transcends all subject–object duality and enables the consequent realization of the elemental emotion. While it is apparent that the eight kinds of rasa[13] have differentiated moods, each welcomed equanimity; the shanta rasa carries the implication of an ultimate emotional state. It is believed that after having experienced the diverse elemental emotional states in an impersonal manner, there is an ultimate quietness, total equanimity.

I wish to emphasize that "rasa" was formerly not a Buddhist concept, yet it consists of equanimity and emptiness in their meditative dimension. For this reason, it may be a useful concept in this discussion. In the context of this chapter, it is depicted as an example of a profound understanding of the essential emotional situations that are void of personal identification. From this perspective, we can assume that the art of rasa illuminates and illustrates higher narcissistic forms and transformations.

This way of presenting elemental emotional states in an impersonal form may also remind us of a Greek chorus that voices the common sense of the people (an ultimate reality). Here, too, expression is given to a supra-individual voice, not a particular one.

If we go back to our discussion of equanimity, we have to emphasize one last point: While some people may regard equanimity as aloofness, neutrality, or indifference, it is in fact a sort of ethical non-attachment of the Bodhisatva and the selfobject that facilitates the empty position. It promotes comprehension of the universal characteristics of emotions and promotes realizing their link to a vast universal interconnectedness. In this sense, equanimity is a dimension of transcendence.

13 The Hindu tradition identifies eight elemental rasas: love, happiness, sorrow, anger, energy, fear, disgust, and astonishment. Each has a characteristic color. Later another rasa was added, the shanta rasa, which consists of stillness and tranquility. Its color is white. It was believed that shanta rasa stems from feelings of despair. It is interesting to note that such feelings were transcended to an experience of tranquility.

Vignette II: Equanimity

A clinical example may illustrate a transcendental transformation of a personal response to terror to an ultimate dimension, using equanimity:

This was a supervision session in a psychoanalytic seminar in Russia. The presenter traveled for ten hours on the bus from a war zone. She presented the following question: "Why is it so hard for me to talk? I want to say things but cannot . . . Why am I crying?" She said that she feels so much anger toward the Kazaks (a minority where she lives) that she cannot accept them as patients. She turns them away. She was very upset and concerned about the ethical implications of her conduct.

She proceeded to describe a female patient, 32 years old. The patient came in wearing a torn dress; her body was shaking, and there was fear in her eyes. The patient explained that she was captured and kept as a hostage during the bloodshed fights between different ethnic groups. The therapist went on to describe her own situation: "I felt numbness. . . . I suggested that she see a doctor . . . she pauses. Since then, I cannot see Kazak patients."

I asked if she could share more about what she feels in regard to the Kazaks. The therapist burst into tears and told me that she had a close friend. One day, the Kazaks caught her son and killed him. The friend found him beheaded at her doorstep.

At this point, I experienced confusion between horrifying fantasies and a dreadful reality. In my mind, the reality and the fantasies were totally intermingled, with no clear boundary between them. I tried to remind myself that I am an "old timer" in regard to trauma and pain and that I have heard so much before. And yet I was speechless. I looked around in the room. There were tears in all eyes. Terror was reflected in everybody's face. Nobody could say a word. I got up and sat next to this therapist and put my hand on hers.

The time was over. She was surrounded by four other women in the group. I saw that they had gone out. I realized that they went directly to the swimming pool area, where the music was on all day and started to dance. They must have danced together for half an hour. The next day, she asked for another meeting to discuss her feelings further privately.

This experience remained in my mind as an extremely powerful illustration of transforming individual terror into a shared, equanimous experience.

In "The Place of Compassion in Political Conflict" (Mann, 2010),[14] I described a situation that developed between a politically left-wing psychotherapist and a patient who was a settler from the West Bank and extremely right-wing. The supervision process led to a transformation from initial dread, contempt, and a wish not to know the patient to a transcendental mode of interconnectedness. I emphasized how such a mode consists of compassion and enables an expansion of the mind.

The supervisee felt that she had lost a precious ideal, her capability to function as an equanimous selfobject to the others. She came to the seminar with the hope of healing this profound wound in her now-split self. She wanted to regain her equanimity, to dissolve/disattach herself from the impact of her personal trauma.

The group process first enabled her to transform individual dread into an experience of shared terror. Holding her hand conveyed my sharing her pain. Consequently, dread was transformed into mental pain. Lastly, the circle of dancing women–mothers–sisters became a channel for the dissolution of sorrow and its transcendence to an ultimate dimension. The dancing provided a non-verbal mode of union, "dancing-out" feelings that could not be spoken about.

A personal trauma was transformed into an experience of interconnectedness. Equanimity became possible when the group functioned as a selfobject and absorbed the personal trauma. They turned an individual trauma into a shared collective experience (Brothers, 2008). This transformation occurred when there was an intuitive realization that suffering is universal and that one is there to experience and share the suffering of the other.

A Final Remark

I hope that this discussion illustrates how the concepts of Boddhisatva, emptiness, and equanimity can inspire and enrich the theory of self psychology and broaden the implications of the selfobject concept. Both self

14 This situation is described in detail Chapter 2. It relates to a therapy that started with intense feelings of contempt because of political tension. Compassion cultivated equanimity and expansion of the mind.

psychology and Buddhism are based on a contextual outlook and share a non-dual perspective. It is believed that one person constitutes the selfhood of the other and is deeply entangled in her process of becoming. In this state of interbeing (Hanh, 2001),[15] we offer ourselves as a receptive "empty other" as best as we can.

These ideas imply that the concept of interbeing offers an elaboration of our common thinking about the selfobject matrix. The selfobject's very presence creates a psychological field comprising non-separable entities. The analyst's emptiness allows for the free emergence of the patient's hidden selfhood with minimal hindrances. In such circumstances, the primordial non-self can emerge.

I wish to close with a quote from the interview[16] Kohut gave to Randall close to his death in April 1981:

> I think that one isn't really alive if one doesn't somehow, down deep in one's bones, feel this eternal rhythm of life, this coming and going of which one is only a link in a chain. . . . It goes beyond my individuality to something broader and more enduring than this little me that is common.

References

Bion, W. R. (1984a). *Second thoughts: Selected papers on psycho-analysis*. Karnac Books.

Bion, W. R. (1984b). *Transformations*. Karnac Books.

Bion, W. R. (1988). Notes on memory and desire. In E. B. Spillius (Ed.), *Melanie Klein today: Developments in theory and practice: Vol. 2: Mainly practice* (pp. 17–21). Routledge.

Brothers, D. (2008). *Toward a psychology of uncertainty: Trauma-centered psychoanalysis*. Analytic Press.

15 Hanh (2001) formulated interbeing as follows: "Formations have the nature of interbeing. The one is produced by the all and the all is dependent on the one." In different terms, self psychologists have written about wholeness (Sucharov, 2013), system theories (Lichtenberg et al., 2011), and complexity theory (Frie & Coburn, 2011), and this is certainly not the full list. All these thinkers convey the idea that broad changeability is induced by interconnected fields, not by particular individuals. American psychoanalysts regard these transformations as relational, while this perspective regards the field as a non-dual entity.

16 See Chapter 7.

Chuang Tzu. (1968). *The complete works of Chuang Tzu* (B. Watson, Trans.). Columbia University Press.

Dōgen. (1994). *Master Dōgen's shobogenzo* (G. Nishijima & C. Cross, Trans.). Windbell Publications.

Eigen, M. (1998). The Unknown Support : Reflections on the Innovations of D. W. Winnicott. *Psychoanalytic Review, 85*(2), 179–198.

Freud, S. (1958). Recommendations to physicians practicing psycho-analysis. In J. Strachley & A. Freud (Eds.), *The standard edition of the complete psychological works of Sigmund Freud: Vol. 12 (1911–1913): The case of schreber papers on technique & other works* (pp. 109–120). Hogarth Press.

Frie, R., & Coburn, W. J. (Eds.). (2011). *Persons in context: The challenge of individuality in theory and practice*. Routledge.

Ghent, E. (2001). Need, paradox, and surrender: Commentary on paper by Adam Phillips. *Psychoanalytic Dialogues, 11*(1), 23–41. https://doi.org/10.1080/10481881109348595

Grotstein, J. S. (2000). *Who is the dreamer who dreams the dream? A study of psychic presences*. Analytic Press.

Hanh, T. N. (2001). *Transformation at the base: Fifty verses on the nature of consciousness*. Parallax Press.

Hanh, T. N. (2022). *Call me by my true names: The collected poems of Thich Nhat Hanh*. Parallax Press.

Kohut, H. (1966). Forms and transformations of narcissism. *Journal of the American Psychoanalytic Association, 14*(2), 243–272. https://doi.org/10.1177/000306516601400201

Kohut, H. (1982). Introspection, empathy, and the semi-circle of mental health. *The International Journal of Psycho-Analysis, 63*(4), 395–407.

Kohut, H. (1984). *How Does Analysis Cure?* eds. A. Goldberg & P. Stepansky. Chicago: University of Chicago Press.

Kohut, H. (1996). *Heinz Kohut: The Chicago institute lectures* (P. Tolpin & M. Tolpin, Eds.). Routledge.

Kulka, R. (1997). Quantum selfhood commentary on paper by Beebe, Lachmann, and Jaffe. *Psychoanalytic Dialogues, 7*(2), 183–187. https://doi.org/10.1080/10481889709539173

Kulka, R. (2012). Between emergence and dissolving: Contemporary reflections on greatness and ideals in Kohut's legacy. *International Journal of Psychoanalytic Self Psychology, 7*(2), 264–285. https://doi.org/10.1080/15551024.2012.656357

Lachmann, F. M. (2007). *Transforming narcissism: Reflections on empathy, humor, and expectations*. Routledge. https://doi.org/10.4324/9780203927267

Lichtenberg, J. D., Lachmann, F. M., & Fosshage, J. L. (2011). *Psychoanalysis and motivational systems: A new look* (pp. xix, 136). Routledge https://doi.org/10.4324/9780203844748

Mann, G. (2007). Emotional blindness and its transformation. *The Psychoanalytic Review, 94*(2), 291–313. https://doi.org/10.1521/prev.2007.94.2.291

Mann, G. (2010, October). *The domain of non-duality: An area of faith.* Presented at the 33rd IAPSP Annual International Conference on the Psychology of the Self, Antalya, Turkey.
Mann, G. (2013). Being human among humans: Response to Maxwell S. Sucharov's "Thoughts on wholeness, connection, and healing: Moving toward complexity in the analytic space". *International Journal of Psychoanalytic Self Psychology*, *8*(4), 398–411. https://doi.org/10.1080/15551024.2013.825946
Mann, G. (2015). The Selfobject Function Revisited: Reaching out beyond the individual. *The International Journal of Psychoanalytic Self Psychology*, *10*(3), 212–223.
Mann, G. (2020). Emptiness, equanimity and the selfobject function. *Psychoanalytic Inquiry*, *40*(5), 300–310. https://doi.org/10.1080/07351690.2020.1766321
Sucharov, M. S. (1992). Quantum physics and self psychology: Toward a new epistemology. In A. I. Goldberg (Ed.), *Progress in self psychology* (Vol. 8, pp. 199–211). Routledge.
Sucharov, M. S. (2013). Thoughts on wholeness, connection, and healing: Moving toward complexity in the analytic space. *International Journal of Psychoanalytic Self Psychology*, *8*(4), 379–397. https://doi.org/10.1080/15551024.2013.825944
Suzuki, S. (1970). *Zen Mind, beginner's mind.* Weatherhill.

Chapter 11

Forms and Transformations of Intergenerational Trauma

Between Oedipus and Odysseus

Introduction

Two Greek myths illustrate the possible means of transformation of intergenerational trauma. One is the myth of Oedipus, and the other is the story of Odysseus. The first, Oedipus, demonstrates a link between the generations while the trauma remains concealed and denied. In contrast, the story of Odysseus exemplifies an intergenerational connection in which intersubjectivity, compassion, and empathy are maintained, together with the fathers' commitment and responsibility for caring for peace among the next generation. A clinical case will illustrate how, in the course of an analysis, the patient was able to make the leap to an Odyssean mode of relating and immersing herself in her natural creativity. As Winnicott (1971) wrote in the chapter "The Location of Cultural Experience":

> In using the word "culture," I am thinking of the inherited tradition. I am thinking of something that is in the common pool of humanity, into which individuals and groups of people may contribute, and from which we may all draw *if we have somewhere to put what we find.*
>
> (p. 99, italics in the original)

Intergenerational trauma has many forms and transformations. In this chapter, I refer to the blind transmission of trauma, which leads to personal and social violence, and the possibility of its transformation. Intergenerational trauma characterizes the experience of many patients I encounter whose parents suffered in different ways during World War II and subsequently. The parents were often victims of prolonged persecution and uprooting. They felt humiliated and ashamed because of what had happened to them and attempted not to subject their children to the tragedies that they had

DOI: 10.4324/9781003449386-11

experienced. They therefore veiled their subjective experiences or falsified them. At the same time, their hushed background permeated the next generation's psyche, often with unconscious violence.

One aspect of such trauma is the brutal rupture created in the relational continuum between the generations. In many cases, intergenerational trauma is an outcome of a desire not to know too much about the first generation's suffering so as to avoid too much mental pain. As a consequence, partial, distorted, or falsified knowledge of one generation about the other's increases. Subjective experiences are erased, concealed, or retold by the traumatized generation in a disjointed way. Thus, the gloomy gap between the generations is packed with true or false projections. They become frozen areas of the mind, areas where the potential for mutual regulation (Lachmann & Beebe, 1996) and emotional intimacy give way to private madness.

My hope is to show that upheavals that occur in the analytic dyad inform and influence the patients' potential for intergenerational transformation. The analytic couple offers an arena for the emergence of entirely unformulated experiences and the opportunity to discover still unexplored relational options. Nonlinear thinking, such as quantum theory, can help in the understanding of such a phenomenon.

Two Greek myths illustrate the possible means of transformation of intergenerational trauma. One is the myth of Oedipus, described in the tragedy of Sophocles, and the other is the story of Odysseus, related in the writings of Homer. The first, Oedipus, demonstrates a link between the generations while the trauma remains concealed and denied. Consequently, Oedipus, the victim of human relationships steeped in denial, is described as blind to the social context in which he lived and lacking compassion toward the other. In contrast, the story of Odysseus exemplifies an intergenerational connection in which intersubjectivity, compassion, and empathy are maintained, together with the fathers' commitment and responsibility for taking care that there be congruence among the next generation.

Oedipus: A Story of Blind Grandiosity

This myth is well known to us all, and there is no need to detail it here. I will just emphasize some points related to the previous generation in this myth that are relevant in the context of this chapter. Oedipus was the son of Laius, king of Thebes. Laius, the father, was cursed by Zeus for raping the son of another king who had sheltered him and later on felt the need to harm him for his transgression. Years later, Laius married Jocasta. When they realized they could not have children, he secretly consulted an oracle and revealed that any child born to him and Jocasta would eventually kill him because of Zeus's curse.

To prevent the prophecy from being realized, Laius distanced himself from Jocasta without disclosing to her the reason. At the height of her distress, Jocasta decided to make her husband drunk and seduce him, which led to Oedipus's birth. It is evident that the couple's tendency to hide the truth was prevalent within the couple's relationship. This chain of events paved the way to perversion.

Following Oedipus's birth, Laius tried to take control of his fate. This belief of his, that he could escape Zeus's prophecy, was an expression of his grandiosity. He shackled the newborn's ankles (hence the name Oedipus, which literally means "swollen foot") and abandoned him to die on the summit of a bare mountain, so hoping to escape from his predicted doom. Oedipus exemplifies an infant suffering the dehumanization of his father. This was the foundation for later hatred, rivalry, and revenge.

The rest of the story is familiar to us. The tragedy ends with Jocasta's suicide, after many years in which she denied the connection between her past and her husband's identity, and Oedipus is blinded after killing his father and going into exile. Oedipus's father's tragedy was transcribed and became Oedipus's fate.

Odysseus: A Story of Idealization and Compassion

When the Greeks began to organize their forces for their campaign against Troy, they mobilized all the kings, their men, ships, and supplies. Odysseus, the king of Ithaca, on the verge of adulthood with a young wife and an infant male offspring, was not at all enthusiastic about going to war. When the envoys of the Greek states came to assess his condition and force him to obey, he feigned illness and pretended to be insane. The messengers found him in a field with an ox and a donkey harnessed together to a saddle. He was throwing salt behind his back and wearing a ridiculous hat, such as is usually worn by the people from the East. He pretended not to recognize his visitors and demonstrated in every way he could think of that he had lost his mind.

But one of the messengers suspected that it was a deception. He grabbed Telemachus, Odysseus's infant son, and hurled him in front of Odysseus's plow. Odysseus instantly turned the plow around in a semicircle to prevent his son from being hurt – an action that immediately revealed the real state of his mental health. Odysseus was forced to admit that he had only pretended to be mad to avoid the journey to Troy. He preferred to live with and be there for his loved ones. This devotion to his family was such an important ideal that, for the sake of its protection, he was willing to pretend to be insane.

Later on, Odysseus went to war and was absent from his home for many years. His wife remained faithful to him, believing that he would return. She waited ten years and rejected numerous suitors. Meanwhile, Odysseus succeeded in conquering Troy, wandering between Troy and other places. He wanted to return to his wife and son, but temptations, dangers, and other obstacles again and again diverted him from getting back to her. Finally, after ten years, he returned to Ithaca. At first, no one recognized him except for his nanny and his faithful dog. Later on, with the help of his son, Telemachus, he proves his identity, kills his wife's suitors, and is accepted as the queen's lost husband and king of Ithaca. The story illustrates the significance and importance of idealized selfobjects.

In the final paper before his death, "Introspection, Empathy and the Semi-Circle of Mental Health," Kohut (1982) tried to summarize his theoretical thinking about humaneness and humanity. He referred to intergenerational ties and their impact on mental health or mental illness. Freudian thinking viewed the drive as the main factor in understanding intergenerational seduction, competitiveness, and destructiveness, as well as the human propensity to kill. Kohut, on the other hand, suggested an alternative paradigm: the parental generation may be obligated to the next generation with pride, warmth, empathy, and joy, thus recognizing its own right to exist, thrive, and differ from the generation that preceded it. For Kohut, being part of the chain of generations is the most meaningful experience a person can have. In such a chain, the young people place themselves shoulder to shoulder alongside their ancestors rather than being their eternal rivals. As Kohut (1982) notes:

> And now a few words about the re-interpretation of the Oedipus myth that I promised you before. It is a remarkable fact that nobody, as far as I know, has pointed out, at least not in an effective way, a feature of the Oedipus myth which refers to the intergenerational relationship – an

aspect of the story, which is truly remarkable, especially by comparison with the parallel aspect of the intergenerational story about Odysseus and Telemachus as told us by Homer. It is as if analysts had reversed their usual stance as regards King Oedipus by taking the manifest content – father murder, incest – as the essence, while disregarding clues, in particular genetic clues, which may allow us to see the relationship between parents and son in a different light. Is it not the most significant dynamic-genetic feature of the Oedipus story that Oedipus was a rejected child? Never mind the all-explanatory oracle that served as a convenient vehicle for rationalizing a human failure as obedience to the gods. The fact is that Oedipus was not wanted by his parents and that he was put out into the cold by them. He was abandoned in the wilderness to die. While his appealing-assertive baby self found substitute parents – down deep the sense of his original rejection must have remained. Does our attention to this part of the story not allow us to see King Oedipus' "Oedipus complex" in a different light? And does it not, by stark contrast, illuminate even further, how Odysseus' normal intergenerational response, the semi-circle of his plough, led to a relationship between father and son – I remind you of their shoulder-to-shoulder fight against outside disturbers, thus re-establishing the interrupted intra-familial bond – which, I submit is the true and nuclear essence of humanness.

(pp. 404–405)

This passage illustrates the way in which Kohut introduced a broad contextual approach influenced by quantum thinking (Sucharov, 1992; Kulka, 1997). The healthy self is aware that it is being formed and transformed by endless changes within its environment. He sees himself as a link in the vast chain of human events. This approach provides a broad view of humanity, which extends beyond the particular individual.

Kohut (1996) raises a significant question: On whom does the main responsibility for this intergenerational disruption fall, on the fathers or on the sons? His response is unequivocal: it is the broken self of the parent or his grandiosity, and not the innocent child, which leads to the maintenance of the trauma. The Laiusian father prefers his own existence and his own good to that of his son. This damaged parental self cannot validate the child's experience of identification in a joyful and empathetic way. Consequently, the infant's self disintegrates and generates hostility and lust.

In his article "On Arrogance," first presented in 1957, Bion (1984, pp. 86–92) suggests that Oedipus's mental position is derived from the child's natural curiosity to know what was going on in his parents' dyadic relationship. When catastrophe lurks beneath the surface, this natural ability is obstructed. The parental container cannot contain the child's curiosity and therefore, instead of constructive curiosity, we meet arrogance, excessive curiosity, and stupidity, signifiers of a human disaster. This disaster is manifest in an "Oedipal mode," an impasse between fathers and sons and deterred intuitive understanding.

This leads us to the question once again: Who was Liaus really? Who was this father who first consciously and then unconsciously confronted his son and wanted to eliminate him? In fact, Liaus was himself a child who was rejected and exiled in his youth and lived under the roof of a king who welcomed him. However, he abducted the king's son and ran away with him. For these acts, Liaus was cursed by the gods and doomed to be killed by any son born to him. This personal tragedy, which can be described as acting out of a fear of a breakdown (Winnicott, 1992, pp. 87–95), led to the unthinkable act of sacrificing his innocent newborn baby, an act indicative of private madness. It was his attempt to erase every trace of his uncanny past and his subjectivity. Laius's narcissistic injury later was expressed in shame and concealment that also concerned his wife, Jocasta. His hidden self was doomed to keep a disastrous secret all to himself.

Under these circumstances he could not find rest for his haunted soul.

We can realize that Oedipus was born into an insecure environment, permeated by pervert tendencies and lacking a dedicated father to secure his safety. His fate was actually informed by the catastrophe of the previous generation. Finally, he took the father's emotional blindness upon himself as a punishment, transformed it into physical blindness, but gained mental lucidity by this act.

In her book *The Telescoping of Generations: Listening to the Narcissistic Links Between Generations*, Haydée Faimberg (2005) describes how a person becomes invisible when they are not being seen or inaudible when they are not listened to. The observer has a direct influence on the object of his observation and the evolution of his subjectivity. In the intergenerational context, objects become "invisible" or "inaudible" when the parental observer relates to them as unworthy of being seen or heard, as irrelevant. Faimberg terms these intergenerational identifications as "alien identifications." She suggests that these identifications are prominent in the Oedipal situation of intergenerational transferences due to the narcissistic logic by which the parent operates, as if to say: what is worthy of recognition is that which resembles me or corresponds to my interests; everything that differs from me is an alien object destined to be hated; if you, my child, will not be similar to me, you will forever be the bearer of all that I repudiate in myself, you will be an other, an object to be hated and rejected.

That is to say that narcissistic parents are internalized as parents who are unable to love their child without appropriating his identity and are incapable of recognizing the child's uniqueness and independence without subjecting him or her to their own experiences of self-hatred. The child becomes a prisoner of his parents' invasiveness. Often, such situations are understood or become meaningful only in retrospect when memories emerge in therapy rather than in real time. Within a therapeutic process, the patient can succeed in discarding these identifications of self within an analysis, with the presence of an idealized selfobject, who promotes the distinctive aspects of the patient's subjectivity.

In the course of these two myths, we learn about the possible relationships between fathers and sons: Odysseus's semicircle is a symbol of the fact that a person whose self is cohesive can experience the next generation as a continuation of his own self, an expression of "being a human among humans" (Kohut, 1984, p. 200). The primacy of supporting the succeeding generation's self is at the forefront of his mind. On the other hand, the story of Oedipus is an allegory for adults who have experienced trauma in their past that cannot be transformed. In working with these people, we must take into account not only the difficulty of the parents' generation to disclose their personal experiences in the analytical process but also the disguised reluctance of the younger generation to discover this knowledge, given the high emotional cost of dealing face to face with the catastrophe that befell their parents. Consciously or unconsciously, the young defend themselves against being the carriers of their parents' transmissions. Conceivably, the comprehension of the trauma exists among them at a certain level, perhaps as intuitive knowledge as "thoughts without a thinker" (Bion, 1984, p. 200) or as the "unthought known" (Bollas, 1987). If we accept this assumption, the unthought known is a meaningful component in the mind.

When thinking about the transformations in the patterns of relating between generations, we have to consider that both generations tend to fluctuate between the "Odyssean mode" and the "Oedipal mode." The first consists of vulnerability, dread, compassion, and mutual regulation. In the second mode, both generations are prone to be defensive and to disregard each other's subjectivity. Instead of living in an environment of shared subjectivity, the self is trapped in a world of deceptions, lies, and riddles.

The Case of Betty[1]

Betty came to therapy harboring harsh feelings about her wasted life. Her wish was to be creative, but she felt unable to create. She had previously experienced a number of disappointing therapies, including a case in which the therapist initiated sexual relations with her. These traumatic events left black holes in her soul.

In one of our first meetings, Betty brought a film she had made years previously. The film, which she called *Sleep*, focused on a girl standing next to a parrot's cage. The girl poked a stick into the parrot's cage to annoy it. The film conveyed an experience of being imprisoned in a tormenting reality devoid of life and hope. What I saw, and particularly the fact that the film was utterly silent, left a strong impression on me. Over time, I learned that under the cover of silence, the patient often experienced moments of madness in which she would discharge her anguish by screaming and banging her head against the wall so as to forget the pain and loneliness she was feeling.

It quite quickly became clear that Betty had been exposed to various traumas in her childhood. One trauma was her mother telling her that she was an unwanted child, "a hole in the diaphragm." Later, she shared intimate events related to her relationship with her husband, such as his betrayals. The patient felt that these facts were rammed into her psyche entirely against her will and without any consideration.

A different trauma arose from her relationship with her father. The father was a 5-year-old boy when World War II broke out. He was on the run for three years with his mother and sister. His survival from the clutches of the Nazis was made possible by his mother's sexual relations with them as well as learning from a young age that survival depends on the ability to manipulate and deceive the environment by presenting a charming and seductive presence. He became the seductive man in Betty's life, very present, very close and, in her experience, often invading her privacy and ignoring her separate existence.

1 The case was published in a different context in Mann (2009).

Betty was disgusted and suffered from these experiences with each of her parents and even realized that she tended to follow similar patterns of behavior herself, especially in her complex relationships with men, including her failed marriage. Our work led us to the understanding that these patterns derived from her mother's failure to endow her with a sense of liveliness and joy. In order not to collapse, she turned her father into an object of desire, an exciting object that provides a sense of vitality, however false it may have been.

Our relationship had its ups and downs. During the initial years of her therapy, Betty found the end of every session and parting from me difficult to cope with. In her imagination, my image was changing and distorted at such times. She was furious when I failed to offer her what she thought she "needed" or when she felt I wasn't sufficiently protective of her. The rage was aimed at me directly, but no less at herself, when she realized the extent to which she was sabotaging her skills and potential, turning opportunities for growth and development into embarrassing sexual experiences that left her naked and empty. "Oops, I'm naked" became the motif that accompanied our work and was used to describe those moments when she turned herself into an object, usually a sexual object, while completely renouncing her experience as a subject. The word "autostrada" also signaled an entry to an area permeated by too many undigested experiences. We realized that these moments indicated unthinkable anxiety.

I invested a great deal of effort deciphering the huge amounts of information that Betty instilled in me verbally as well as through written materials that she gave me. Sometimes, I felt invaded and not even able to properly digest and decipher the full significance of the materials she presented to me. Betty may have allowed me, in this way, to understand something about her inability to decipher various personal experiences in the face of the complex of uncontrolled stimuli that life confronted her with.

One day, after two years of therapy, Betty handed me a folder containing all her communications with me and about me in the context of the analysis: "I don't want to write to you anymore. You keep these materials and from now on we will talk," she announced firmly. I knew that she was responding to the excesses that we often experienced between us and that she was trying to regulate herself so that we would be in sync with one another. I could sense an emerging hope and the belief that we would find the right rhythm and space for better mutual regulation.

One of the recurring narratives was an issue surrounding money. Initially, she asked to pay for the analysis in cash so that I would lower the price, given that she was receiving money from her father for her use. I gently refused this offer and explained to her something about freedom for each of us in the analysis. Then, she raised the question as to when she would be paying for the analysis. Every month, when payment was due, I felt her resentment, frustration, and anger beneath the surface. In the end, she admitted that she felt it was a humiliation for her to pay with the money she was getting from her father, which she considered "unclean." She was afraid that paying with this tainted money would tarnish our relationship and destroy it. The more we delved into thinking about this issue, it became clear that for her, the money issue was evidence of her unspoken consent to her father's intrusion into the most personal aspects of her life.

In one of our sessions, she suddenly shared a new memory: her father was arrested for tax offenses when she was a child. In fact, she had completely forgotten this event and only now, in the analysis, remembered it with horror. Was it right for her to continue to accept her father's methods of financial "survival" without having to be ashamed, without feeling that she is complicit in his actions? In this context, another memory emerged; she used to steal from the nearby grocery store small things like a pack of candy, a toothbrush. . . . Was she a liar, or was she a victim of her loneliness and emptiness, a girl with no one with whom she could share her sadness? At that point, she realized that her difficulties with money, including her past tendency to steal, were connected to a kind of secrecy and obfuscation common within the family, as well as a life-saving strategy.

One of the main issues that accompanied our work was how to find a way to deal with her father's constant seductiveness/invasiveness. Her father used to tell her about various medical problems and took pains to expose parts of his body "to show her." He used to offer to go shopping together and then start flirting with the saleswoman, which made her want to disappear and, if possible, be erased completely so as not to be part of the embarrassing situation. These events made her feel so uncomfortable.

Gradually, the nature of the relationship with her father became increasingly clearer. The relationship was largely based on the link between money and sexuality, her subjection to a Faustian contract according to which whatever she would receive from him would be contingent on agreeing to his excessive intrusion and consent to be humiliated and abused. This clear observation of the link between these issues gradually reduced their traumatic impact and allowed a more compassionate approach to them.

In the fourth year, after a vacation, we had the following exchange:

B: I see his aggression and let it happen. When my response is softened, his aggression doesn't develop. It makes room for something else between us. To feel the love.
G: His touch, now, is not too close.
B: It is different. He shares with me things related to his life, his work, aging friends.
G: A wide range of mutual concerns.

And later, in a trembling voice:

B: I understand how important your presence, your being here with me, is to me. When you weren't there, I was so pressured that I couldn't hold on to the love for him. You explained that it happens when there are too many things going on and no one is there. . . . I've been mentally killing you for the past few weeks. I turned you into something unreal; I couldn't believe I'd be back here, on the couch.
G: When I'm not here, there are holes in our relationship.

The next day, when she arrived, she covered herself with the knitted blanket she always used and said:

> I was thinking about yesterday. . . . You mentioned holes in our relationship and I thought about the holes in the blanket. . . . There is a blanket. But there are holes in the blanket.

G: Sometimes you feel the blanket, and sometimes you feel the holes.
B: That's true, but what's important is that there are holes in *this* blanket. This blanket allowed me to cope with holes and not run away.
G: With *this* blanket, holes don't pursue you.
B: The roof won't fall on me. . . . I've been through a lot of suffering in my life, by accident or not [she cries]. We worked hard to get *this* far, and what's most important: *this* is my blanket . . . my wrapping.
G: One can endure a hole when it is in the blanket.

B: In the past, there was only a hole. There was no blanket. That's why I ran away. You asked if I worked in your absence. No. It is impossible to be creative when there is no blanket.

I thought about the black holes in her mind, which she mentioned at the beginning of our journey. In their invasive patterns, each of her parents violently dug holes in Betty's psyche. Her mother rammed her with inappropriate information, and her father pierced her psyche with his boundless sexuality. These holes in her mind became signifiers of disaster areas, evidence of intergenerational trauma. They were drilled into her mind by Oedipal parents who prioritized self-preservation over nurturing the peace of their children. During the analysis, these black holes were gradually transformed into "holes in the blanket," holes between threads, and finally when the traumatic experiences were transformed, they evolved into potential spaces.

Simultaneously with our work on the relationship with her parents, Betty was concerned about her relationship with her daughter. She felt she had nothing to offer, and her daughter distanced herself from her. As the analysis progressed, Betty realized that she might lose her daughter if she continued to be increasingly unresponsive to her needs.

The following is another excerpt from an analytical session after a vacation. At that time, her daughter was enlisting in the army, and her father was planning a vacation.

B: He [her father] doesn't say that the plan for a trip suits him but implies that the plan would be good for me. A little lie. . . . I know very well how he activates other people. I grew up with these tricks. There is something paralyzing about these manipulations, when something is turned into something else.

G: And you are supposed to accept it even if you recognize it as a lie.

B: Yes, and it is also expected of me to give him a bonus for something you didn't get. I remember all kinds of small incidents like that.

G: Small distortions are sometimes more hurtful than big ones, maddening lies.

B: You know [silence], as a child, I clutched at every crumb of love and had to express gratitude for being so lucky. Only now can I hear and identify the endless noise, this confusion. One has to lose one's mind.

> And the main thing – no recognition of who I am, what my talents are, my writing. They didn't care that I was an excellent student. This is the difficulty of my life, I failed to value myself.
> [silence]
> In the last three weeks, when you weren't here, something happened. You went on your trip, and I went on mine. With my daughter! This time, I did something different; I discovered that I could live.
> In Barcelona, things started to get confused. I called you once and left a message. I just wanted to hear your voice on the answering machine, but you answered. That was enough. I have no words. My daughter has a different mother. I'm not like my mother.

Having a safety blanket supporting her, she could now think in a lucid way and give up repetitions of past patterns in front of her children; she was able to discover for herself new ways of how to live a different life.

This quiet place opened up an opportunity for a prolonged and gentle deciphering of the possible links between mothers and daughters, daughters, and fathers, both through discourse about her daughter and through her transference to me as her analytic mother. Our work became more and more focused and uninterrupted; we could communicate with less noise and more precision. I learned to notice the pace of her steps down the path toward my clinic. I knew when she was nervous, sad, or happy, even before she lay down on the couch. What was important at this stage was micro-interactions between us, tiny oscillations of mutual being. The tone becomes almost more significant than the content.

Over time, Betty learned to listen to me in a similar way.

One day, she realized within the hour that she was not properly prepared for an important professional meeting. The next day, she asked: "Why did you swing your leg at the end of yesterday's meeting?" and continued:

> I used to think that when you move your leg like that, you are angry with me . . . making a motion of kicking me. This time again I saw you move your leg, but I thought you were moving because you were nervous for me. You move your leg when I screw up.

I realized that Betty now saw the movement of my leg as an indicator of *her* state of being. At this point, Betty could consider the possibility that the other not only is self-centered but contains her distress *for her*. I felt that this moment was precious and special, maybe a kind of "now moment." Betty experienced, even if for just momentarily, the possibility of merging to an experience of non-duality, a mode of being that is beyond common interaction.

In the fifth year, the bulk of our work revolved around Betty's creative work and its development. At the beginning of the analysis, writing served the function of a healing selfobject in the absence of a living subject to support her. Writing allowed a compulsive repudiation of her agony, just as my computer was used to store her distressing materials. The mute and tolerant paper served as an infinite container.

As the analysis went on, Betty discovered a growing interest in professional writing and began writing short stories. By implication, she let me understand that the stories were about me and us. I tried to minimize my reactions to these stories based on my understanding that her creativity was emerging, and this process should be allowed to happen without hindrance.

The subject of creativity became an agonizing and exhausting matter and led to a feeling of being stumped. I recognized my involvement in her writing and its link to my father who so wanted me to become a writer. I realized that I was developing too much "desire" to help her when she should be coping with her difficulties by finding the right content as well as a resolution to the question of whether she really has enough creativity and if she really wants to be a writer. I mentioned that we should think about the possibility that she wouldn't become a writer. I needed to hold this possibility in my mind and allow it to be.

In the next meeting, she entered the room and surprised me with her clear words:

> When I was so lonely, I wrote instead of living. I was so transparent that I could only sustain myself through stories. You touched on the central question: whether I can truly immerse myself in writing or is this another lie? In this sense, writing is the most accurate mirror there is.

At this point, the patient was in the process of publishing her third book. Her relationship with her father had undergone a marked change. She shared with him her everyday experiences with ease and joy. She traveled with him to his hometown in Poland and illustrated the compassion that she discovered toward him in a short story about the trip:

> During my stay with my father, it seemed to me that I had forgotten my age, my previous relationships, and the roles I had taken on. In Krakow, I was just my father's daughter. I asked him questions, I listened, we laughed, had fun, and felt the pain. I tried to understand his needs, as well as myself. . . . What does it mean to be my father's daughter?

From Private Madness to a Context of Compassion

The recovery of the mind is a process of participating with the patient in their courageous attempt to witness the trauma of the previous generation – its consequences for them – and their daring to share the pain of this generation without falling victim to its fate. Dissociations and vertical splits can become experiences of integration and even unintegration and take on new meanings. In the midst of such transformation, patients may show empathy for the wounded psyche of the parents. Private madness evolves into a context of compassion.

Communication with the analyst is a process that increases the cohesion of the self in the sense that something amorphous takes shape through continuous listening, recognition, and validation of detached states of self (Bromberg, 2006). The analyst listens carefully to the subtle fluctuations between the patient's willingness to know and the need not to know. When the analyst recognizes a potential for wishing to know, she tries to adopt reflective communication with those parts. This is how the subjectivity of the patient is established.

Here, I mean not only the unconscious material and its transformation into the conscious mind but also the concealed parts of the self that were known and not recognized. In the right emotional context, these hidden elements of the self can emerge, be seen, and be heard. What was invisible becomes visible; what was inaudible becomes audible. The full potential can be realized in a healthier and more cohesive self. Under such conditions, the patient can experience relationships they had never experienced before. In this sense, we are not dealing with the analysis of transference as a repetition. Rather, we are dealing with selfobject transferences for the purpose of a shared construction of experiences that have not been previously endured.

The presence of the analyst should be such that the patient feels safe enough to dare and experience in the analytic context what has not been experienced before (Winnicott, 1992, pp. 87–95). From this point, communication will be established. The very fact that there is such a presence, an alternative to alien identifications, may lead to the old defensive wall dissolving. This transformation may stimulate a yearning to continue to examine additional gaps of information, such as improbable family stories and lies that have not yet been touched upon. It is the courage to confront the shameful parts of the psyche without having to split them off or project them into the psyches of others. We are talking about nonlinear transformations that occur in tiny segments of mutual regulation.

Return to the Clinical Case

A tragic Oedipal mode became an Odyssean mode of mutual existence and connection. Because she could listen to her father, be close to him, and position herself shoulder to shoulder with him, an intra-family bond was created, a context of compassion (Kohut, 1966; Orange, 2006). Betty could perceive her pain in relation to her father as related to his past and to the deprivation he suffered from rather than viewing it as evidence that he did not care about her. In this sense, she could finally comprehend her private madness as a tragic fate shared by many children of traumatized parents. There is no doubt that it is a tragedy that such children do not get the opportunity in life to thrive as they deserve. However, in the right context, they can bring about changes and transformations.

The clinical case illustrates how the father's unresolved Oedipal traumas were projected into his daughter's psyche. Since he was unable to assimilate his own traumas and detoxify them, he projected them onto his daughter, who was unable to decipher the meaning of these traumas, as she herself had not experienced them. Only when these toxic substances were dissolved in the analysis could this patient choose to be her father's daughter out of her own free will and not under coercion. For the same reason, she could then become a writer, out of her ideal self and not out of attachment to writing as a defensive structure.

At this point we can ask: What enables the patient who grew up in an Oedipal matrix to make the leap to an Odyssean mode? What is there in the analysis that enables this change? I believe that the opportunity to experience selfobject transferences in an analysis, and interconnection in the relation with the analyst, is what leads to this opportunity to have a new beginning. This means that not only do we put an end to unfortunate repetitions, but we also help the patient to become a different parent, a different person, another son or daughter, who exists in an Odyssean mode.

This understanding frees the patient and removes from her the burden of shame and vulnerability. The patient can be more empathic toward her own disavowed self-states when there is no longer a need to follow the confusing expectations of the previous generation. The vulnerability diminishes, replaced by mature narcissism, which allows one to relate to the tragic fate of others. It makes it possible for a member of one generation to become an active partner in the suffering of the previous damaged generation and take full responsibility for the well-being of the next generation. This is what made it possible for Betty to cultivate her creative skills.

I would like to add one comment: we should all, as analysts, pay close attention to our "Oedipal" moments, as opposed to our "Odyssean" moments. The Oedipal places are those where we involve our own self-interest, our self-cherishing motives, where we sometimes abandon our patients and leave them to face their fate alone. Such situations in analysis are not only a sign of the return of what was repressed but evidence of our significant personal traumas that restrict the mind.

References

Bion, W. (1984). *Second thoughts: Selected papers on psycho-analysis*. Karnac Books.

Bollas, C. (1987). *The shadow of the object: Psychoanalysis of the unthought known*. Columbia University Press.

Bromberg, P. M. (2006). *Awakening the dreamer: Clinical journeys*. Analytic Press.

Faimberg, H. (2005). *The telescoping of generations: Listening to the narcissistic links between generations*. Routledge.

Kohut, H. (1966). Forms and transformations of narcissism. *Journal of the American Psychoanalytic Association, 14*(2), 243–272. https://doi.org/10.1177/000306516601400201

Kohut, H. (1982). Introspection, empathy, and the semi-circle of mental health. *The International Journal of Psycho-Analysis*, *63*(4), 395–407.

Kohut, H. (1984). *How does analysis cure?* (A. Goldberg & P. Stepansky, Eds.). University of Chicago Press.

Kohut, H. (1996). *Heinz Kohut: The Chicago institute lectures* (P. Tolpin & M. Tolpin, Eds.). Routledge.

Kulka, R. (1997). Quantum selfhood: Commentary on paper by Beebe, Lachmann, and Jaffe. *Psychoanalytic Dialogues*, *7*(2), 183–187. https://doi.org/10.1080/10481889709539173

Lachmann, F. M., & Beebe, B. (1996). The contribution of self- and mutual regulation to therapeutic action: A case illustration. In A. I. Goldberg (Ed.), *Progress in self psychology: Vol. 12: Basic ideas reconsidered* (pp. 123–140). Routledge.

Mann, G. (2009). Between submission, surrender and dissolving – Beyond intersubjectivity. *The Israeli Journal of Psychotherapy "Sihot"*, *23*, 161–169.

Orange, D. M. (2006). For whom the bell tolls: Context, complexity, and compassion in psychoanalysis. *International Journal of Psychoanalytic Self Psychology*, *1*(1), 5–21. https://doi.org/10.2513/s15551024ijpsp0101_2

Sucharov, M. (1992). Quantum Physics and Self Psychology. *Progress in Self Psychology*, *8*, 199–211.

Winnicott, D. W. (1971). *Playing and reality*. Basic Books.

Winnicott, D. W. (1992). *Through paediatrics to psycho-analysis: Collected papers*. Karnac Books.

Index

Note: Page numbers in *italic* indicate a figure on the corresponding page.